# STNA
## Exam

# SECRETS

## Study Guide
Your Key to Exam Success

**STNA Test Review for the**
**State Tested Nursing Assistant Exam**

Dear Future Exam Success Story:

First of all, **THANK YOU** for purchasing Mometrix study materials!

Second, congratulations! You are one of the few determined test-takers who are committed to doing whatever it takes to excel on your exam. **You have come to the right place.** We developed these study materials with one goal in mind: to deliver you the information you need in a format that's concise and easy to use.

In addition to optimizing your guide for the content of the test, we've outlined our recommended steps for breaking down the preparation process into small, attainable goals so you can make sure you stay on track.

We've also analyzed the entire test-taking process, identifying the most common pitfalls and showing how you can overcome them and be ready for any curveball the test throws you.

Standardized testing is one of the biggest obstacles on your road to success, which only increases the importance of doing well in the high-pressure, high-stakes environment of test day. Your results on this test could have a significant impact on your future, and this guide provides the information and practical advice to help you achieve your full potential on test day.

Your success is our success

**We would love to hear from you!** If you would like to share the story of your exam success or if you have any questions or comments in regard to our products, please contact us at **800-673-8175** or **support@mometrix.com**.

Thanks again for your business and we wish you continued success!

Sincerely,
The Mometrix Test Preparation Team

**Need more help? Check out our flashcards at:** http://MometrixFlashcards.com/STNA

# TABLE OF CONTENTS

# Introduction

**Thank you for purchasing this resource**! You have made the choice to prepare yourself for a test that could have a huge impact on your future, and this guide is designed to help you be fully ready for test day. Obviously, it's important to have a solid understanding of the test material, but you also need to be prepared for the unique environment and stressors of the test, so that you can perform to the best of your abilities.

For this purpose, the first section that appears in this guide is the **Secret Keys**. We've devoted countless hours to meticulously researching what works and what doesn't, and we've boiled down our findings to the five most impactful steps you can take to improve your performance on the test. We start at the beginning with study planning and move through the preparation process, all the way to the testing strategies that will help you get the most out of what you know when you're finally sitting in front of the test.

We recommend that you start preparing for your test as far in advance as possible. However, if you've bought this guide as a last-minute study resource and only have a few days before your test, we recommend that you skip over the first two Secret Keys since they address a long-term study plan.

If you struggle with **test anxiety**, we strongly encourage you to check out our recommendations for how you can overcome it. Test anxiety is a formidable foe, but it can be beaten, and we want to make sure you have the tools you need to defeat it.

# Secret Key #1 – Plan Big, Study Small

There's a lot riding on your performance. If you want to ace this test, you're going to need to keep your skills sharp and the material fresh in your mind. You need a plan that lets you review everything you need to know while still fitting in your schedule. We'll break this strategy down into three categories.

## Information Organization

Start with the information you already have: the official test outline. From this, you can make a complete list of all the concepts you need to cover before the test. Organize these concepts into groups that can be studied together, and create a list of any related vocabulary you need to learn so you can brush up on any difficult terms. You'll want to keep this vocabulary list handy once you actually start studying since you may need to add to it along the way.

## Time Management

Once you have your set of study concepts, decide how to spread them out over the time you have left before the test. Break your study plan into small, clear goals so you have a manageable task for each day and know exactly what you're doing. Then just focus on one small step at a time. When you manage your time this way, you don't need to spend hours at a time studying. Studying a small block of content for a short period each day helps you retain information better and avoid stressing over how much you have left to do. You can relax knowing that you have a plan to cover everything in time. In order for this strategy to be effective though, you have to start studying early and stick to your schedule. Avoid the exhaustion and futility that comes from last-minute cramming!

## Study Environment

The environment you study in has a big impact on your learning. Studying in a coffee shop, while probably more enjoyable, is not likely to be as fruitful as studying in a quiet room. It's important to keep distractions to a minimum. You're only planning to study for a short block of time, so make the most of it. Don't pause to check your phone or get up to find a snack. It's also important to **avoid multitasking**. Research has consistently shown that multitasking will make your studying dramatically less effective. Your study area should also be comfortable and well-lit so you don't have the distraction of straining your eyes or sitting on an uncomfortable chair.

The time of day you study is also important. You want to be rested and alert. Don't wait until just before bedtime. Study when you'll be most likely to comprehend and remember. Even better, if you know what time of day your test will be, set that time aside for study. That way your brain will be used to working on that subject at that specific time and you'll have a better chance of recalling information.

Finally, it can be helpful to team up with others who are studying for the same test. Your actual studying should be done in as isolated an environment as possible, but the work of organizing the information and setting up the study plan can be divided up. In between study sessions, you can discuss with your teammates the concepts that you're all studying and quiz each other on the details. Just be sure that your teammates are as serious about the test as you are. If you find that your study time is being replaced with social time, you might need to find a new team.

# Secret Key #2 – Make Your Studying Count

You're devoting a lot of time and effort to preparing for this test, so you want to be absolutely certain it will pay off. This means doing more than just reading the content and hoping you can remember it on test day. It's important to make every minute of study count. There are two main areas you can focus on to make your studying count:

## Retention

It doesn't matter how much time you study if you can't remember the material. You need to make sure you are retaining the concepts. To check your retention of the information you're learning, try recalling it at later times with minimal prompting. Try carrying around flashcards and glance at one or two from time to time or ask a friend who's also studying for the test to quiz you.

To enhance your retention, look for ways to put the information into practice so that you can apply it rather than simply recalling it. If you're using the information in practical ways, it will be much easier to remember. Similarly, it helps to solidify a concept in your mind if you're not only reading it to yourself but also explaining it to someone else. Ask a friend to let you teach them about a concept you're a little shaky on (or speak aloud to an imaginary audience if necessary). As you try to summarize, define, give examples, and answer your friend's questions, you'll understand the concepts better and they will stay with you longer. Finally, step back for a big picture view and ask yourself how each piece of information fits with the whole subject. When you link the different concepts together and see them working together as a whole, it's easier to remember the individual components.

Finally, practice showing your work on any multi-step problems, even if you're just studying. Writing out each step you take to solve a problem will help solidify the process in your mind, and you'll be more likely to remember it during the test.

## Modality

*Modality* simply refers to the means or method by which you study. Choosing a study modality that fits your own individual learning style is crucial. No two people learn best in exactly the same way, so it's important to know your strengths and use them to your advantage.

For example, if you learn best by visualization, focus on visualizing a concept in your mind and draw an image or a diagram. Try color-coding your notes, illustrating them, or creating symbols that will trigger your mind to recall a learned concept. If you learn best by hearing or discussing information, find a study partner who learns the same way or read aloud to yourself. Think about how to put the information in your own words. Imagine that you are giving a lecture on the topic and record yourself so you can listen to it later.

For any learning style, flashcards can be helpful. Organize the information so you can take advantage of spare moments to review. Underline key words or phrases. Use different colors for different categories. Mnemonic devices (such as creating a short list in which every item starts with the same letter) can also help with retention. Find what works best for you and use it to store the information in your mind most effectively and easily.

# Secret Key #3 – Practice the Right Way

Your success on test day depends not only on how many hours you put into preparing, but also on whether you prepared the right way. It's good to check along the way to see if your studying is paying off. One of the most effective ways to do this is by taking practice tests to evaluate your progress. Practice tests are useful because they show exactly where you need to improve. Every time you take a practice test, pay special attention to these three groups of questions:

- The questions you got wrong
- The questions you had to guess on, even if you guessed right
- The questions you found difficult or slow to work through

This will show you exactly what your weak areas are, and where you need to devote more study time. Ask yourself why each of these questions gave you trouble. Was it because you didn't understand the material? Was it because you didn't remember the vocabulary? Do you need more repetitions on this type of question to build speed and confidence? Dig into those questions and figure out how you can strengthen your weak areas as you go back to review the material.

Additionally, many practice tests have a section explaining the answer choices. It can be tempting to read the explanation and think that you now have a good understanding of the concept. However, an explanation likely only covers part of the question's broader context. Even if the explanation makes sense, **go back and investigate** every concept related to the question until you're positive you have a thorough understanding.

As you go along, keep in mind that the practice test is just that: practice. Memorizing these questions and answers will not be very helpful on the actual test because it is unlikely to have any of the same exact questions. If you only know the right answers to the sample questions, you won't be prepared for the real thing. **Study the concepts** until you understand them fully, and then you'll be able to answer any question that shows up on the test.

It's important to wait on the practice tests until you're ready. If you take a test on your first day of study, you may be overwhelmed by the amount of material covered and how much you need to learn. Work up to it gradually.

On test day, you'll need to be prepared for answering questions, managing your time, and using the test-taking strategies you've learned. It's a lot to balance, like a mental marathon that will have a big impact on your future. Like training for a marathon, you'll need to start slowly and work your way up. When test day arrives, you'll be ready.

Start with the strategies you've read in the first two Secret Keys—plan your course and study in the way that works best for you. If you have time, consider using multiple study resources to get different approaches to the same concepts. It can be helpful to see difficult concepts from more than one angle. Then find a good source for practice tests. Many times, the test website will suggest potential study resources or provide sample tests.

## Practice Test Strategy

If you're able to find at least three practice tests, we recommend this strategy:

1.  Take the first test with no time constraints and with your notes and study guide handy. Take your time and focus on applying the strategies you've learned.
2.  Take the second practice test open-book as well, but set a timer and practice pacing yourself to finish in time.
3.  Take any other practice tests as if it were test day. Set a timer and put away your study materials. Sit at a table or desk in a quiet room, imagine yourself at the testing center, and answer questions as quickly and accurately as possible.
4.  Keep repeating step 3 on a regular basis until you run out of practice tests or it's time for the actual test. Your mind will be ready for the schedule and stress of test day, and you'll be able to focus on recalling the material you've learned.

# Secret Key #4 – Pace Yourself

Once you're fully prepared for the material on the test, your biggest challenge on test day will be managing your time. Just knowing that the clock is ticking can make you panic even if you have plenty of time left. Work on pacing yourself so you can build confidence against the time constraints of the exam. Pacing is a difficult skill to master, especially in a high-pressure environment, so **practice is vital**.

Set time expectations for your pace based on how much time is available. For example, if a section has 60 questions and the time limit is 30 minutes, you know you have to average 30 seconds or less per question in order to answer them all. Although 30 seconds is the hard limit, set 25 seconds per question as your goal, so you reserve extra time to spend on harder questions. When you budget extra time for the harder questions, you no longer have any reason to stress when those questions take longer to answer.

Don't let this time expectation distract you from working through the test at a calm, steady pace, but keep it in mind so you don't spend too much time on any one question. Recognize that taking extra time on one question you don't understand may keep you from answering two that you do understand later in the test. If your time limit for a question is up and you're still not sure of the answer, mark it and move on, and come back to it later if the time and the test format allow. If the testing format doesn't allow you to return to earlier questions, just make an educated guess; then put it out of your mind and move on.

On the easier questions, be careful not to rush. It may seem wise to hurry through them so you have more time for the challenging ones, but it's not worth missing one if you know the concept and just didn't take the time to read the question fully. Work efficiently but make sure you understand the question and have looked at all of the answer choices, since more than one may seem right at first.

Even if you're paying attention to the time, you may find yourself a little behind at some point. You should speed up to get back on track, but do so wisely. Don't panic; just take a few seconds less on each question until you're caught up. Don't guess without thinking, but do look through the answer choices and eliminate any you know are wrong. If you can get down to two choices, it is often worthwhile to guess from those. Once you've chosen an answer, move on and don't dwell on any that you skipped or had to hurry through. If a question was taking too long, chances are it was one of the harder ones, so you weren't as likely to get it right anyway.

On the other hand, if you find yourself getting ahead of schedule, it may be beneficial to slow down a little. The more quickly you work, the more likely you are to make a careless mistake that will affect your score. You've budgeted time for each question, so don't be afraid to spend that time. Practice an efficient but careful pace to get the most out of the time you have.

# Secret Key #5 – Have a Plan for Guessing

When you're taking the test, you may find yourself stuck on a question. Some of the answer choices seem better than others, but you don't see the one answer choice that is obviously correct. What do you do?

The scenario described above is very common, yet most test takers have not effectively prepared for it. Developing and practicing a plan for guessing may be one of the single most effective uses of your time as you get ready for the exam.

In developing your plan for guessing, there are three questions to address:

- When should you start the guessing process?
- How should you narrow down the choices?
- Which answer should you choose?

## When to Start the Guessing Process

Unless your plan for guessing is to select C every time (which, despite its merits, is not what we recommend), you need to leave yourself enough time to apply your answer elimination strategies. Since you have a limited amount of time for each question, that means that if you're going to give yourself the best shot at guessing correctly, you have to decide quickly whether or not you will guess.

Of course, the best-case scenario is that you don't have to guess at all, so first, see if you can answer the question based on your knowledge of the subject and basic reasoning skills. Focus on the key words in the question and try to jog your memory of related topics. Give yourself a chance to bring the knowledge to mind, but once you realize that you don't have (or you can't access) the knowledge you need to answer the question, it's time to start the guessing process.

It's almost always better to start the guessing process too early than too late. It only takes a few seconds to remember something and answer the question from knowledge. Carefully eliminating wrong answer choices takes longer. Plus, going through the process of eliminating answer choices can actually help jog your memory.

Summary: Start the guessing process as soon as you decide that you can't answer the question based on your knowledge.

# How to Narrow Down the Choices

The next chapter in this book (**Test-Taking Strategies**) includes a wide range of strategies for how to approach questions and how to look for answer choices to eliminate. You will definitely want to read those carefully, practice them, and figure out which ones work best for you. Here though, we're going to address a mindset rather than a particular strategy.

Your chances of guessing an answer correctly depend on how many options you are choosing from.

| How many choices you have | How likely you are to guess correctly |
| --- | --- |
| 5 | 20% |
| 4 | 25% |
| 3 | 33% |
| 2 | 50% |
| 1 | 100% |

You can see from this chart just how valuable it is to be able to eliminate incorrect answers and make an educated guess, but there are two things that many test takers do that cause them to miss out on the benefits of guessing:

- Accidentally eliminating the correct answer
- Selecting an answer based on an impression

We'll look at the first one here, and the second one in the next section.

To avoid accidentally eliminating the correct answer, we recommend a thought exercise called **the $5 challenge**. In this challenge, you only eliminate an answer choice from contention if you are willing to bet $5 on it being wrong. Why $5? Five dollars is a small but not insignificant amount of money. It's an amount you could afford to lose but wouldn't want to throw away. And while losing $5 once might not hurt too much, doing it twenty times will set you back $100. In the same way, each small decision you make—eliminating a choice here, guessing on a question there—won't by itself impact your score very much, but when you put them all together, they can make a big difference. By holding each answer choice elimination decision to a higher standard, you can reduce the risk of accidentally eliminating the correct answer.

The $5 challenge can also be applied in a positive sense: If you are willing to bet $5 that an answer choice *is* correct, go ahead and mark it as correct.

Summary: Only eliminate an answer choice if you are willing to bet $5 that it is wrong.

# Which Answer to Choose

You're taking the test. You've run into a hard question and decided you'll have to guess. You've eliminated all the answer choices you're willing to bet $5 on. Now you have to pick an answer. Why do we even need to talk about this? Why can't you just pick whichever one you feel like when the time comes?

The answer to these questions is that if you don't come into the test with a plan, you'll rely on your impression to select an answer choice, and if you do that, you risk falling into a trap. The test writers know that everyone who takes their test will be guessing on some of the questions, so they intentionally write wrong answer choices to seem plausible. You still have to pick an answer though, and if the wrong answer choices are designed to look right, how can you ever be sure that you're not falling for their trap? The best solution we've found to this dilemma is to take the decision out of your hands entirely. Here is the process we recommend:

Once you've eliminated any choices that you are confident (willing to bet $5) are wrong, select the first remaining choice as your answer.

Whether you choose to select the first remaining choice, the second, or the last, the important thing is that you use some preselected standard. Using this approach guarantees that you will not be enticed into selecting an answer choice that looks right, because you are not basing your decision on how the answer choices look.

This is not meant to make you question your knowledge. Instead, it is to help you recognize the difference between your knowledge and your impressions. There's a huge difference between thinking an answer is right because of what you know, and thinking an answer is right because it looks or sounds like it should be right.

Summary: To ensure that your selection is appropriately random, make a predetermined selection from among all answer choices you have not eliminated.

# Test-Taking Strategies

This section contains a list of test-taking strategies that you may find helpful as you work through the test. By taking what you know and applying logical thought, you can maximize your chances of answering any question correctly!

It is very important to realize that every question is different and every person is different: no single strategy will work on every question, and no single strategy will work for every person. That's why we've included all of them here, so you can try them out and determine which ones work best for different types of questions and which ones work best for you.

## Question Strategies

### Read Carefully

Read the question and answer choices carefully. Don't miss the question because you misread the terms. You have plenty of time to read each question thoroughly and make sure you understand what is being asked. Yet a happy medium must be attained, so don't waste too much time. You must read carefully, but efficiently.

### Contextual Clues

Look for contextual clues. If the question includes a word you are not familiar with, look at the immediate context for some indication of what the word might mean. Contextual clues can often give you all the information you need to decipher the meaning of an unfamiliar word. Even if you can't determine the meaning, you may be able to narrow down the possibilities enough to make a solid guess at the answer to the question.

### Prefixes

If you're having trouble with a word in the question or answer choices, try dissecting it. Take advantage of every clue that the word might include. Prefixes and suffixes can be a huge help. Usually they allow you to determine a basic meaning. Pre- means before, post- means after, pro - is positive, de- is negative. From prefixes and suffixes, you can get an idea of the general meaning of the word and try to put it into context.

### Hedge Words

Watch out for critical hedge words, such as *likely, may, can, sometimes, often, almost, mostly, usually, generally, rarely*, and *sometimes*. Question writers insert these hedge phrases to cover every possibility. Often an answer choice will be wrong simply because it leaves no room for exception. Be on guard for answer choices that have definitive words such as *exactly* and *always*.

### Switchback Words

Stay alert for *switchbacks*. These are the words and phrases frequently used to alert you to shifts in thought. The most common switchback words are *but, although,* and *however*. Others include *nevertheless, on the other hand, even though, while, in spite of, despite, regardless of*. Switchback words are important to catch because they can change the direction of the question or an answer choice.

## Face Value

When in doubt, use common sense. Accept the situation in the problem at face value. Don't read too much into it. These problems will not require you to make wild assumptions. If you have to go beyond creativity and warp time or space in order to have an answer choice fit the question, then you should move on and consider the other answer choices. These are normal problems rooted in reality. The applicable relationship or explanation may not be readily apparent, but it is there for you to figure out. Use your common sense to interpret anything that isn't clear.

# Answer Choice Strategies

## Answer Selection

The most thorough way to pick an answer choice is to identify and eliminate wrong answers until only one is left, then confirm it is the correct answer. Sometimes an answer choice may immediately seem right, but be careful. The test writers will usually put more than one reasonable answer choice on each question, so take a second to read all of them and make sure that the other choices are not equally obvious. As long as you have time left, it is better to read every answer choice than to pick the first one that looks right without checking the others.

## Answer Choice Families

An answer choice family consists of two (in rare cases, three) answer choices that are very similar in construction and cannot all be true at the same time. If you see two answer choices that are direct opposites or parallels, one of them is usually the correct answer. For instance, if one answer choice says that quantity $x$ increases and another either says that quantity $x$ decreases (opposite) or says that quantity $y$ increases (parallel), then those answer choices would fall into the same family. An answer choice that doesn't match the construction of the answer choice family is more likely to be incorrect. Most questions will not have answer choice families, but when they do appear, you should be prepared to recognize them.

## Eliminate Answers

Eliminate answer choices as soon as you realize they are wrong, but make sure you consider all possibilities. If you are eliminating answer choices and realize that the last one you are left with is also wrong, don't panic. Start over and consider each choice again. There may be something you missed the first time that you will realize on the second pass.

## Avoid Fact Traps

Don't be distracted by an answer choice that is factually true but doesn't answer the question. You are looking for the choice that answers the question. Stay focused on what the question is asking for so you don't accidentally pick an answer that is true but incorrect. Always go back to the question and make sure the answer choice you've selected actually answers the question and is not merely a true statement.

## Extreme Statements

In general, you should avoid answers that put forth extreme actions as standard practice or proclaim controversial ideas as established fact. An answer choice that states the "process should be used in certain situations, if..." is much more likely to be correct than one that states the "process should be discontinued completely." The first is a calm rational statement and doesn't even make a definitive, uncompromising stance, using a hedge word *if* to provide wiggle room, whereas the second choice is a radical idea and far more extreme.

## Benchmark

As you read through the answer choices and you come across one that seems to answer the question well, mentally select that answer choice. This is not your final answer, but it's the one that will help you evaluate the other answer choices. The one that you selected is your benchmark or standard for judging each of the other answer choices. Every other answer choice must be compared to your benchmark. That choice is correct until proven otherwise by another answer choice beating it. If you find a better answer, then that one becomes your new benchmark. Once you've decided that no other choice answers the question as well as your benchmark, you have your final answer.

## Predict the Answer

Before you even start looking at the answer choices, it is often best to try to predict the answer. When you come up with the answer on your own, it is easier to avoid distractions and traps because you will know exactly what to look for. The right answer choice is unlikely to be word-for-word what you came up with, but it should be a close match. Even if you are confident that you have the right answer, you should still take the time to read each option before moving on.

# General Strategies

## Tough Questions

If you are stumped on a problem or it appears too hard or too difficult, don't waste time. Move on! Remember though, if you can quickly check for obviously incorrect answer choices, your chances of guessing correctly are greatly improved. Before you completely give up, at least try to knock out a couple of possible answers. Eliminate what you can and then guess at the remaining answer choices before moving on.

## Check Your Work

Since you will probably not know every term listed and the answer to every question, it is important that you get credit for the ones that you do know. Don't miss any questions through careless mistakes. If at all possible, try to take a second to look back over your answer selection and make sure you've selected the correct answer choice and haven't made a costly careless mistake (such as marking an answer choice that you didn't mean to mark). This quick double check should more than pay for itself in caught mistakes for the time it costs.

## Pace Yourself

It's easy to be overwhelmed when you're looking at a page full of questions; your mind is confused and full of random thoughts, and the clock is ticking down faster than you would like. Calm down and maintain the pace that you have set for yourself. Especially as you get down to the last few minutes of the test, don't let the small numbers on the clock make you panic. As long as you are on track by monitoring your pace, you are guaranteed to have time for each question.

**Don't Rush**

It is very easy to make errors when you are in a hurry. Maintaining a fast pace in answering questions is pointless if it makes you miss questions that you would have gotten right otherwise. Test writers like to include distracting information and wrong answers that seem right. Taking a little extra time to avoid careless mistakes can make all the difference in your test score. Find a pace that allows you to be confident in the answers that you select.

**Keep Moving**

Panicking will not help you pass the test, so do your best to stay calm and keep moving. Taking deep breaths and going through the answer elimination steps you practiced can help to break through a stress barrier and keep your pace.

# Final Notes

The combination of a solid foundation of content knowledge and the confidence that comes from practicing your plan for applying that knowledge is the key to maximizing your performance on test day. As your foundation of content knowledge is built up and strengthened, you'll find that the strategies included in this chapter become more and more effective in helping you quickly sift through the distractions and traps of the test to isolate the correct answer.

Now it's time to move on to the test content chapters of this book, but be sure to keep your goal in mind. As you read, think about how you will be able to apply this information on the test. If you've already seen sample questions for the test and you have an idea of the question format and style, try to come up with questions of your own that you can answer based on what you're reading. This will give you valuable practice applying your knowledge in the same ways you can expect to on test day.

Good luck and good studying!

# Safety

## Preventing Patient Falls

Patient falls are a considerable problem in the health care setting. Injuries resulting from a fall are considered to be a primary cause of morbidity in older adults. The loss of coordination and bone density as people age puts them at an increased risk for breaking bones after a fall; the resultant loss of independence may lead to a decline in health and eventual death. Yet falling is not a normal part of aging. Proper prevention can greatly decrease a patient's risk of falling. As a nurse aide, it is important to follow fall precautions to prevent patient falls within the hospital setting.

### Precautions

There are a number of precautions that can be taken to prevent patient falls. The first step of prevention is identifying the needs of the patient. If the patient has been determined to be a fall risk, a sign should be placed on the door so the staff knows the patient has special mobility needs. While the patient is in bed, at least two side rails should be kept in the raised position to prevent the patient from falling out of bed. Prior to standing with assistance, patients should be allowed to sit or dangle at the side of the bed to prevent dizziness that may result from the change in position. The patient should also wear rubber-soled shoes or socks.

The floor should be kept free of all hazards, including puddles of water and small rugs that can cause slipping. While the patient sits in or stands up from the chair or wheelchair, the brakes should be kept locked.

## Bed-Bound Patient

Patients who are bedridden have a particularly high risk of falling.

While the patient is in bed, make sure the side rails are up to prevent the patient from climbing out of bed. If necessary, a bed alarm may be placed in the bed to alert the nurse aide that the patient is attempting to get out of bed without assistance.

The patient's call light should be placed within reach, as well as the patient's tray table and any other items the patient might need. Toileting should be offered at least every two hours, and the patient should be turned every two hours to prevent bedsores.

## Transferring the Patient

Patient strength should be assessed prior to moving the patient to determine how much assistance may be required.

While the patient is in bed, make sure the brakes are locked and the bed is in the lowest position. Lower the side rail, and raise the head of the bed until it is at a comfortable level for the patient.

While facing the patient, place one arm behind the shoulders and one arm beneath the knees. Assist the patient into a sitting position at the side of the bed. Allow the patient to remain there for a few moments to ensure the patient is not dizzy from the change in position.

*Transferring patient from a bed to a wheelchair:* Care must be taken while transferring a patient from the bed to the wheelchair to prevent falling during the transfer.

Prior to moving the patient, make sure the bed and wheelchair wheels are locked to prevent movement during ambulation.

Ensure the patient is wearing rubber-soled socks or shoes to prevent slipping. Make sure the patient is not suffering from any dizziness or lightheadedness that may result from a quick change in position. Prior to beginning the transfer, explain the procedure to the patient.

*Procedure for transferring patient from a bed to a wheelchair:* Move the wheelchair as close to the bed as possible, and make sure the wheels are locked. Lift the leg pads and footplates up and out of the way to prevent tripping. Explain the procedure to the patient.

Assist the patient into a dangling position. Place your feet in a wide stance. Instruct the patient to stand on the count of three, and support the torso while helping the patient into a standing position. Pivot the patient so that his back is to the wheelchair. Instruct the patient to position his arms on the armrests of the wheelchair and back up until he feels the seat against the backs of his legs. Slowly lower the patient into a sitting position. Assist the patient in lifting his legs and placing the leg pads and footplates beneath them.

*Procedures for transferring the patient from bed to a stretcher:* While the patient is lying in bed, make sure the wheels of the bed and the stretcher are locked. Raise the level of the bed until it is the same height as the stretcher. If available, a slider board can be placed beneath the patient to facilitate movement and decrease friction.

Stand at the side of the stretcher, and ask a colleague to stand next to the bed. Instruct the patient to cross his arms over his chest to prevent dragging his limbs across the bed. Grasp the draw sheet, and roll it to maintain a good grip. On the count of three, pull the draw sheet toward you, while the colleague at the side of the bed pushes the patient from the other side. Continue to pull until the patient is in the center of the stretcher. Position the patient for comfort.

## Types of Assistance

Stand by Assistance (SBA), Contact Guard Assistance (CGA), Minimum (MIN), and Maximum (MAX) assistance refer to the level of assistance the patient requires while ambulating.

A patient who can move independently requires SBA. This patient does not require any assistance in ambulating and does not require a gait belt.

CGA refers to a patient who does not require assistance but is at risk for falling. The nursing aide should be close enough to touch the patient in case he should fall, but does not provide additional support.

MIN assistance refers to the patient who needs a small amount of support while ambulating. A gait belt is advised for this type of patient.

Patients who require MAX assistance may or may not be able to bear their own weight. This type of patient requires support from one or two staff members to ensure that he does not fall.

## Falling with a Patient

Even with all necessary precautions properly observed while ambulating, the patient is still at risk for falling. A fall may result if the patient's legs give out from under him or if he were to lose consciousness while ambulating. If a sudden fall were to occur, it is important to protect the patient and yourself from harm.

Support the patient using the gait belt and your free arm, and gently lower the patient to the floor or to a nearby chair, taking care to protect the patient's head. If the fall is uncontrolled as a result of loss of balance, focus on supporting the patient as much as possible while keeping you safe. Try to avoid tensing up prior to impact as this may cause additional injury.

**Patient on Crutches**

The four-point technique is the preferred method of ambulation for a patient with poor lower body strength who is ambulating with crutches.

While the patient is standing, instruct him to move the left crutch forward first, followed by the right foot. The right crutch should then be moved forward, followed by the left foot. The advantage of this method of ambulation is that the patient has at least three points of contact with the ground at all times, offering the most stability; the disadvantage is that it requires a slow movement speed.

The three-point technique is recommended for patients who are unable to bear weight on one foot while ambulating with crutches. While in a standing position, the patient should move both crutches and the affected limb forward. Then, while placing his weight on the crutches, the patient should move his strong leg forward until it is even with the affected extremity.

Swing-to method and the swing-through method of ambulation: The swing-to and swing-through methods of crutch walking are intended for patients who have decreased lower body strength. Both methods are advantageous in that they are easy to learn and allow for a quick gait. The disadvantage is that both methods require strong upper body strength.

In the swing-to method, both crutches are moved forward and placed at the length of a step in front of them. The patient then places his weight upon the crutches and swings his body forward until his feet are equal to the crutches. In the swing-through method, both crutches are moved forward. Placing his weight upon the crutches, the patient swings his lower body forward and places his feet slightly in front of the crutches.

*How a crutch should fit a patient:* Though it is the job of the physical therapist to adjust crutches properly to the size of the patient, the crutch should be checked prior to each ambulation to make sure it continues to fit properly.

The pads of the crutch should remain one to one-and-a-half inches below the axillary area. The handgrips should be even with the patient's hips. When the patient is in a standing position with hands resting on the handgrips, his elbows should be slightly flexed.

When the patient walks on crutches, he should support his weight with his hands on the handgrips. Placing his weight on the pads in the axillary area may cause nerve damage. The patient should keep the head and shoulders erect to limit back strain and keep the torso aligned with the crutches to prevent loss of balance and injury.

*Transfer a patient from a chair or sitting position to a standing position using crutches:* While the patient is sitting in the chair: Instruct him to hold both crutches in one hand by gripping the handgrips. Instruct the patient to scoot his hips to the edge of the chair and stretch the non-weight-bearing foot out straight. Help the patient rise to a standing position, using the arm of the chair to support one of the patient's arms and the crutches to support the other. Once the patient has balanced his weight on one foot, instruct the patient to move one of the crutches to the opposite side and place his hands on the handgrips.

*Transfer a patient from a standing to a sitting position using crutches:* To move from a standing to a sitting position: Instruct the patient to approach the chair until he is one step away from the front of the chair. Instruct the patient to carefully turn using his weight-bearing leg and the crutches until his back is to the chair. Assist the patient in finding his balance before transferring one of the crutches to the opposite side. Instruct the patient to grip both crutches by the handgrips. Help the patient to reach back with his free hand to find the arm of the chair. Instruct the patient to stretch the non-weight-bearing foot in front of him. Assist the patient with slowly lowering his weight into the chair.

## Patient Wearing a Cast

Patients who are wearing a cast must be monitored closely to ensure they have continued circulation.

If the fingers or toes of the extremity with the cast become cool, pale, or bluish in color, these findings should be reported to the nurse immediately.

Sudden severe pain, numbness, or tingling may be an indication of poor circulation or nerve damage and should also be reported.

A foul smell or a burning sensation coming from beneath the cast may be an indication of infection, which should immediately be reported.

## Patient with a Cane

While ambulating a patient who is learning how to walk with a cane, always provide the patient with a gait belt.

Instruct the patient to hold the cane in his strong hand. As the patient takes a step forward with the affected extremity, advance the cane forward, keeping the cane even with the leg and the patient's full weight upon his strong leg. Once the weakened leg and the cane are in place, instruct the patient to place his weight upon the cane while taking a step forward with the unaffected extremity. Allow the patient a moment to regain his balance before repeating the process.

## Patient with a Walker

A patient, who is learning to ambulate with a walker, should wear a gait belt at all times.

Instruct the patient to stand in the middle of the walker, holding it by the handgrips. Instruct the patient to move the walker forward until the back legs are even with the toes. While keeping his weight on the strong leg, the patient should then take a step forward with the weaker leg, until it is in the center of the walker. Then, instruct the patient to place his weight upon the handgrips while taking a step forward with his strong leg. Once he has regained his balance, repeat the process.

*Procedure for assisting a patient from a sitting position to standing with a walker:* While the patient is sitting in the chair, open the walker and place it in front of him. Make sure the patient is wearing a gait belt. Instruct the patient to scoot forward until he is sitting on the edge of the chair. Instruct the patient to place both hands on the arms of the chair. On the count of three, assist the patient into a standing position. While providing support for the patient, instruct him to move his hands, one at a time, from the arms of the chair to the handgrips of the walker. Wait a moment to ensure the patient is not dizzy before beginning to ambulate.

## Safety During Ambulation

While the patient is ambulating, make sure to provide support using a gait belt. Ensure the patient is wearing rubber-soled slippers. If the patient is receiving oxygen therapy, obtain a rolling tank so the patient can continue to wear oxygen while ambulating. Carefully monitor the patient's respirations, and frequently check to make sure the patient is not becoming fatigued or dizzy. Move at a pace that is comfortable for the patient, and do not try to rush him. If necessary, allow the patient to stop to take a brief rest in a chair to ensure that he does not become overexerted.

## Oxygen Administration

There are a number of precautions that should be taken to ensure the patient's safety while receiving oxygen therapy. The patient should be carefully monitored to ensure he is on an appropriate amount of oxygen. The patient and family members should be reminded of the facility's no smoking policy, as oxygen is highly flammable.

Petroleum-based products should not be used while the patient is on oxygen, as these are also highly flammable. Care should be taken to make sure the patient does not become entangled in the oxygen tubing. Oxygen tanks should be stored in their appropriate holders; an oxygen tank can cause serious harm if it were to be knocked over and damaged.

## Unresponsive Patient

Time is of the essence in treating a patient who is found unresponsive. If the patient is unarousable, call for help immediately. Check for breathing by leaning close to the patient's nose and mouth, listening for breath sounds, and watching for the rise and fall of the chest. If the patient is not breathing, administer two rescue breaths using an Ambu bag. Then check the patient's pulse. If the patient does not have a pulse, it is important to initiate CPR as quickly as possible. Lower the head of the bed, and place a backboard beneath the patient to ensure adequate compressions. Follow BLS protocols while attempting to revive the patient.

## Silently Choking

Only initiate the Heimlich maneuver if the patient is conscious but unable to speak or make noise as this indicates that he is choking. Move behind the patient and wrap your arms around them. Make a fist with one hand and place it against the patient's abdomen with the thumb about 2 inches above the umbilicus. Wrap your other hand around your fist. Thrust your fist in and upward with as much force as possible. Continue to do this until the object has been dislodged from the airway or until the patient loses consciousness.

## Ensure Fire Safety

Fire safety is very important in both the hospital and extended-care facility. Because of the presence of highly flammable materials, such as oxygen tanks, proper fire safety must be closely observed.

The nurse aide should make note of the presence of oxygen shutoff valves, fire alarms, and fire extinguishers, and know the facility policy regarding fire alarms. Regular fire drills should be performed, and residents should be aware of necessary fire safety precautions. The fire extinguishers should be serviced regularly to ensure proper functioning. The nurse aide should also be aware of the facility code that indicates a fire. Though a fire is typically announced as a Code Red on the overhead speakers, individual facilities may have different alarm codes.

## RACE

RACE is an acronym that explains the proper procedure that should be performed upon discovery of a fire within the hospital or extended-care facility.

The letter R stands for rescue. The first priority is to remove any patients who are in immediate danger from the fire. The nurse aide should only attempt to rescue a patient if she can do so without placing herself in imminent danger.

The letter A stands for alert. Once any patients have been removed from danger, the nurse aide should activate the fire alarm system, if it has not already been done.

The letter C stands for contain. Fire doors should be closed in an attempt to deprive the fire of oxygen.

The letter E stands for extinguish. If it is safe to do so, attempt to extinguish the fire using the appropriate fire extinguisher.

## PASS

PASS refers to the proper way to handle a fire extinguisher.

The letter P stands for pull. A plastic ring keeps the fire extinguisher from being discharged accidentally. Pull the plastic ring off the fire extinguisher to ready it.

The letter A stands for aim. Aim the nozzle of the fire extinguisher at the base of the fire.

The first S stands for squeeze. Squeeze the trigger of the fire extinguisher to start the flow.

The second S stands for sweep. Sweep the nozzle from side to side, covering the area of the fire completely. Continue to aim at the base of the fire, and do not stop the flow of fluid until the fire has been extinguished.

## Fire Extinguishers

There are three types of fire extinguishers that are typically found in a hospital or extended-care facility.

1. Type A fire extinguisher; it is typically silver in color and shoots pressurized water. Type A fire extinguishers are intended for ordinary combustibles, such as paper, wood, or cloth.
2. Type C fire extinguisher; shoots dry chemicals. It is typically red in color and is intended for fires started from an electrical source, such as a frayed wire or a piece of faulty equipment.
3. Type ABC or multipurpose fire extinguisher. These are also red in color and are intended for fires that have been started by either a combustible, liquid chemical or electrical source.

Before using a fire extinguisher, it is important to make note of which type you are using; a Type A fire extinguisher should not be used on an electrical fire.

## Emergency Treatment for Burns

Depending on the severity and the amount of body surface it covers, a burn can be a life-threatening injury. Shock induced by a burn and the resultant impairment of the immune system can cause serious harm to the patient.

It is important to act quickly if the patient has been severely burned. A burn that extends over a small area of the body should be treated by running cool water over the affected area. A sterile dressing should be applied over the burn to protect the skin and to prevent the introduction of germs. Ice packs should also be applied to protect the skin and nerve endings.

## Electrical Safety

Proper electrical safety is an important step in fire prevention. The maintenance department should regularly service all patient care equipment.

The nursing aide should regularly check to make sure that all equipment is within its maintenance period. If a piece of equipment appears to be malfunctioning, it should be removed from service immediately. Prior to a piece of equipment of being used, it should be checked carefully to make sure its wires are intact. When plugging in a piece of equipment, make sure the circuits are not being overloaded. Also, closely monitor the floor near a piece of equipment to make sure there are no puddles nearby.

## Good Body Mechanics

Proper body mechanics are described as the safe completion of tasks by using the appropriate muscle groups in order to avoid straining or injury. Health care workers have the highest incidences of work-related muscle injuries as a result of frequent heavy lifting, and these injuries are often slow to heal. Proper body mechanics are important in the medical field because of the frequent need to lift, turn, and reposition patients. Good body mechanics ensure the avoidance of using back muscles while caring for the patient, resulting in decreased fatigue and reduced risk of injury for both the patient and the nurse aide.

### Principles of Proper Body Mechanics

There are four principles of body mechanics that should be followed in order to avoid injury.

1. The first is to maintain a proper center of gravity. This is done by bending and lifting with the legs and keeping your back straight as you are lifting.
2. The second principle of body mechanics is to maintain a wide base of support, in order to maintain stability while lifting. Establish this wide base of support by keeping your feet at least 12 inches apart, with one foot slightly ahead of the other.
3. The third principle is to maintain proper alignment. While lifting a heavy object, keep your back straight and the item that you are lifting close to you. If you need to turn with the object, pivot your whole body rather than twisting with the object.
4. The fourth principle of body mechanics is to maintain proper posture while lifting. Keep your head up, your back straight, your knees flexed, and your buttocks tucked in to prevent injury while lifting.

## Moving the Patient Up in the Bed

Never try to move a patient up in bed by yourself. Always ask another nursing aide or nurse to help you. Prior to moving the patient up in bed, explain to the patient what you are going to do.

- Wash your hands, and don a pair of gloves.
- Lay the head of the bed as flat as possible, and raise the level of the bed until it is a comfortable height for you.
- Position yourself near the head of the bed on one side, while the other person moves to the opposite side of the bed.

- Instruct the patient to cross his arms over his chest to prevent his limbs from dragging and to tuck his chin to his chest. If the patient is unable to do so, support the back of his neck with one hand.
- Grasp the draw sheet and roll the edge to establish a good grip.
- On the count of three, lift the draw sheet and pull upward.
- Position the patient for comfort.

## Patient Restraints

Restraint policies vary from one facility to another, but their purpose remains the same.

Restraints are applied in order to protect the patient from causing harm to himself or to other people. A restraint may be applied to prevent the patient from interfering with medical devices or moving in a way that would be detrimental to his health. It may also be applied if the patient is showing signs of aggression. A restraint should always be applied after all other alternatives have been exhausted.

It should not be applied as a form of punishment or for the convenience of the staff.

*Different types of restraints:* There are a number of different types of restraints that can be used in a health care setting.

- Emotional restraints are a method of using verbal or emotional cues in order to attempt to modify the patient's behaviors. This can include limit setting or contracting with the patient for safety.
- Environmental restraints are devices used to restrict patient movement. These include side-rails on the bed or locked doors within the facility. When all four side-rails are in a raised position on the bed, it is considered to be a restraint.
- Physical restraints are devices that can be applied to the patient to restrict movement. These include wrist and vest restraints, lap belts, and movement pads.
- Chemical restraints are medications that are given to the patient to modify behavior.

*Alternatives that must be pursued prior to the application of restraints:* There are a number of measures that can be performed as an alternative to applying restraints. The type of alternatives that are utilized may vary depending upon the patient. Any needs should be assessed and all reasonable alternatives performed prior to application of restraints.

The patient may need to be moved to a quiet environment. He may require more stimulation, such as hearing a television or radio in the background. He may require redirection. The patient may need toileting or water. He may need personal items placed within reach. He may require distraction if the care team is attempting to remove a medical device. If the patient has an illness or requires rest, it may cause him to act in a manner that is confused or inappropriate.

*Prior to applying restraints to the patient:*
all other alternatives must be exhausted. The health care staff must attempt to identify and address the behaviors that require the application of restraints.

An order from the patient's physician must be obtained in order to apply restraints, and the physician should visibly assess the patient within 24 hours of the time of application of the restraints.

Consent should be obtained from the patient's next of kin. Care must be taken to choose the least restrictive form of restraint. The type of restraint should be explained to the patient, as well as the reasons for the application of the restraint and the requirements for removal of the restraint.

*Applying a vest restraint procedure;* the vest restraint is a device that is placed over the patient's chest to restrict their movement. It is typically applied to prevent a patient from getting up without assistance. A doctor's order and consent from the family must be obtained prior to application of the restraint.

- The nurse aide should wash her hands and don a pair of gloves.
- She should greet the patient and explain the need for the restraint, as well as the requirements for removal.
- The vest restraint should be placed on the patient so that the opening is toward the back, with the straps crossing in the back.
- The straps should then be tied with a quick release knot directly to the chair or the frame of the bed.
- At least two fingers should be able to fit beneath the vest restraint to ensure that it is not too tight.
- Once the restraint has been applied, remove the gloves and wash your hands.
- Monitor the patient per facility policy.

*Applying restraints to the extremities:*

Extremity restraints are applied to the arms and legs to restrict movement. A doctor's order and consent from the family must be obtained prior to application of these restraints.

- The nurse aide should wash her hands and don a pair of gloves.
- She should greet the patient and explain the need for the restraint, as well as the requirements for removal.
- The restraint should be applied per the manufacturer's instructions and tied to the frame of the bed using a quick release knot.
- The patient should be given a reasonable amount of slack in order to move.
- The nurse aide should be able to fit two fingers between the patient's extremity and the restraint; this ensures that is it not too tight.

*Securing restraints to a wheelchair versus a bed:* When securing restraints on a patient who is in a wheelchair, care should be taken to ensure the restraint is tied using a quick release knot attached directly to the frame of the wheelchair. The wheelchair should be locked, and care should be taken to ensure the restraints are not tied to the wheels.

- When the patient is in bed, the restraint should be tied using a quick release knot attached directly to the frame of the bed. Tying the restraint to the side rail can cause injury to the patient if the side rail should fall.

*Proper procedure for monitoring a patient who is in restraints:* Patients who are in restraints should be closely monitored to ensure safety.

- They should be checked every 30 minutes to make sure there is proper circulation.
- While they are restrained, patients should have their legs covered with a blanket in order to maintain privacy.
- The restraint should be removed every 2 hours to allow for range of motion.

- Patients should also be repositioned for comfort and offered water and toileting every two hours.
- Teaching regarding the restraints should be frequently reinforced to encourage patient understanding of the need for the restraint and the requirements for removal.

# Infection Control

## Hand Washing

Microorganisms are present on all surfaces and can be transferred via touch. Certain microorganisms can cause illness or infection if they come into contact with a person whose immune system has been compromised. As a result, hand washing is a vital part of infection control. If properly done, hand washing removes visible dirt and germs from the hands. It prevents transmission of germs from the nurse aide to the patient or from one patient to another patient. Warm water, antimicrobial soap, and firm friction applied to all areas of the hand while washing are all key factors in ensuring that the hands are clean and free of germs.

*Hand washing procedures:*
- Before beginning to wash, remove any jewelry on your hands.
- Run the water until it is warm, and then wet hands to the wrist.
- Apply a small amount of soap.
- Continue to work the soap into lather for at least 30 seconds, using firm friction between the fingers, underneath the fingernails, and up the wrists.
- Make sure to keep your hands lower than the elbows to prevent germs from traveling up the arm.
- If your hands have been soiled with body fluids, hand washing should be performed for at least one minute.
- Rinse hands thoroughly with warm water, and then dry your hands.
- When your hands are dry, use part of the towel to turn the faucet off.

*Hand washing should be performed:* frequently to prevent transmission of germs.

- The nurse aide should wash her hands prior to eating, after going to the bathroom, or after sneezing.
- The aide should also wash her hands prior to feeding the patient, before performing any procedures with the patient and after the procedure is complete.
- Hand washing should be performed after coming into contact with a patient's wound, with soiled linen, or with any patient body fluids, even if the nurse aide was wearing gloves at the time.
- The nurse aide should also wash her hands prior to leaving the patient's room.

Proper hand washing is the key to infection control. Because germs run off the hands while hand washing is performed, it is important to ensure that hands do not touch the inside of the sink while washing.

If a nurse aide's hands touch the inside of the sink, then hand washing should be repeated to ensure her hands have not become contaminated.

*Washing with bar soap:* a wet surface of bar soap can provide a medium for germs to grow:

- Prior to beginning to wash hands, rub the soap vigorously to remove the outermost layer of soap.
- Then, once hand washing has been completed, rinse the soap with warm water.

*Cleansing hands with alcohol scrub:* hand sanitizers have been approved as an adjunct to hand washing in the health care setting. They work by removing the outer layer of oils on the hand, killing any bacteria on the hand in the process.

- To use alcohol scrub, take a dime-sized amount into your dominant hand.
- Rub your hands together vigorously for at least thirty seconds.
- Make sure to rub between your fingers, between your knuckles, and beneath the fingernails.
- If, after thirty seconds, your hands are still damp, allow them to air dry.
- Once your hands have dried, they are considered clean.

*Alcohol scrub versus hand washing:* though hand sanitizer has been approved as an adjunct for hand washing, it was not intended to replace it. There are instances in which hand washing is preferred over use of an alcohol-based hand sanitizer.

A nurse aide should wash her hands if they have been soiled with secretions. Hand washing should be used prior to eating and after using the bathroom. Even if hand sanitizer is used, hands should occasionally be washed to remove any residue that can build up as a result of frequent use of alcohol scrub.

## Isolation

Isolation refers to special measures taken to prevent the spread of germs. The goal is to protect other patients and hospital staff while providing care to the patient. Isolation may be required if the patient has a particularly infectious disease, such as tuberculosis or Varicella. The patient may also be placed into isolation if he has a drug-resistant bacterium, such as methicillin-resistant staphylococcus aureus (MRSA) or clostridium difficile (C. diff). Depending upon the type of isolation, the nurse aide may be required to wear an isolation gown, gloves, or a mask while providing care for the patient.

### Types

There are three types of isolation.

1. Contact precautions are intended to limit the spread of microorganisms that might be transmitted by direct contact with a contaminated surface. If a patient is in contact isolation, he should be in a private room that is clearly marked. When providing care to the patient, the nurse aide should wear an isolation gown and gloves at all times while in the room.
2. Droplet precautions are intended to limit the spread of microorganisms that are transmitted via mucous or respiratory secretions. A patient who requires droplet precautions should be placed in a private room. A nurse aide should wear a mask and gloves when caring for a patient who is in droplet precautions.
3. Airborne precautions are intended to prevent the spread of airborne microorganisms that can survive for long periods of time in the environment. While on airborne precautions, the patient should be placed in a negative pressure room. While caring for the patient, the nurse aide should wear a mask or respirator and gloves.

### Items for a Patient in Isolation

The nursing aide should take care to ensure that germs from a patient in isolation are not spread amid the patient population.

A cart should be placed outside of the patient's room containing isolation equipment that should be donned prior to entering the room. This includes waterproof isolation gowns, gloves, and masks, as well as a garbage bag for waste disposal. Germicidal wipes should also be available to clean the equipment that must be shared with the rest of the patient population. The patient in isolation can also be provided with disposable equipment that might ordinarily be shared among the patient population, such as single-use stethoscopes and blood pressure cuffs.

## Personal Protective Equipment (PPE)

Gloves are the most commonly used piece of protective equipment in the health care setting. They are typically made of thin vinyl or nitrile rubber and are intended for single use. They should be used whenever there is a risk of touching infectious material or body fluids.

Gowns are typically made of thin plastic or synthetic waterproof fibers. They are typically worn over the uniform whenever the patient is in contact isolation.

Face protection falls into two categories.

1. Facemasks are worn over the nose and mouth to prevent inhalation of infectious material.
2. Goggles are worn over the eyes to prevent introduction of infectious materials to the eyes.

When dealing with a copious amount of secretions, a face shield can be worn in place of a facemask and goggles.

## Isolation Gown, Gloves, and Mask & Removal

Isolation equipment should be donned before entering an isolation room. The gown should be unfolded and held with the opening toward your back. Place your arms through the sleeves. Tie the gown securely behind the neck and at the waist. Then, put on the facemask, making sure your nose and mouth are covered. Gloves should be applied last and worn so they cover the cuffs of the isolation gown.

Isolation gear should be removed prior to leaving the room. The gloves should be removed first. Grasp the first glove at the wrist and pull to remove it. Then ball the used glove in the hand that is still gloved. Grasp the remaining glove at the wrist and pull to remove it. Next, remove the gown and the mask. Once the gloves, gown, and mask have been removed, wash your hands.

### Removal of Soiled Linen

Care must be taken while removing soiled linen from an isolation room. Because the linen bag was in the isolation room, it is considered contaminated. The soiled linen bag must be placed inside a clean bag to prevent contamination.

While the nursing aide is bathing the patient, soiled linen should be placed in a plastic linen bag. Once bathing has been completed, the linen bag should be tied securely shut. Another aide standing outside the door should hold a second linen bag open while the first bag is placed inside; the second bag should also be tied securely shut. The double-bagged linen bag should be left outside while the nurse aide removes her isolation gown, gloves, and mask, and washes her hands. Then, the soiled linen can be taken to the soiled utility room.

*Precautions to take to prevent the spread of microorganisms while changing linens:*
While removing dirty linens, the nurse aide should wear gloves and avoid holding them close to her body.

Soiled linens should not be shaken out as this may release germs into the air. Once all of the soiled linens have been removed from the bed and put into the appropriate receptacle, the nurse aide should remove her gloves and wash her hands. She should then securely tie the linen bag closed and place it in the soiled utility room. Clean linens should be carefully unfolded and placed on the bed. Any linen that has fallen on the floor should be considered contaminated; it should be placed in the soiled utility bin and replaced with clean linen.

## Universal Precautions

Universal precautions involve treating all patient secretions as if they contain a pathogen, resulting in the avoidance of direct contact with any secretions. Universal precautions are practiced in the health care setting whenever there is the risk of coming into contact with blood or body fluids. The precautions include wearing gloves when collecting blood or handling anything that may have been contaminated with blood. Use of other protective equipment may be necessary, such as wearing a face shield when suctioning copious secretions or a facemask to protect oneself from airborne secretions. If blood or body fluids have contaminated a work surface, it should be cleaned using the appropriate disinfectant.

Cleaning refers to the process that removes visible dirt or soiled material from a surface. It typically involves using water or a detergent to rinse the surface. Cleaning must be performed prior to disinfection or sterilization.

Disinfection is defined as the process that destroys most microorganisms on the surface of a piece of equipment. The disinfectant that is used is typically chemical in nature, though some pieces of equipment may be disinfected using heat.

Sterilization refers to the process that removes all forms of microbial life from a piece of equipment.

## Patient Care Equipment Infection Risk

The level of risk for infection refers to the likelihood that a piece of equipment will contain infectious pathogens on its surface; it aids in determining the proper level of cleaning prior to subsequent use.

Low-risk or noncritical items are pieces of equipment that come into contact with intact skin, such as stethoscopes. Noncritical items also include inanimate objects in the environment, such as countertops and walls. These items only require cleaning with a detergent prior to subsequent use.

Intermediate-risk items are those that come in close contact with mucous membranes but do not penetrate the skin, such as thermometers or respiratory equipment. These items require cleaning with a high-level disinfectant before they are ready for use.

High-risk items, such as surgical instruments and devices, have penetrated the skin and are at high risk for contamination by microorganisms. These items require sterilization before they are ready for subsequent use.

## Cleaning Equipment Steps

Cleaning refers to the process of removing dirt or organic material from the surface of a piece of equipment. If an item is not properly cleaned, subsequent disinfection or sterilization may not be effective. Gloves should be worn while cleaning equipment. Thoroughly wipe each piece of equipment with a detergent, rubbing with firm pressure to remove any dirt or organic material.

Once the organic material and dirt has been removed, rinse the surface thoroughly with water and allow it to dry prior to subsequent use. Hand washing should be performed after cleaning any equipment.

*Steps for sterilizing equipment:* Sterilization requires a piece of equipment be exposed to extreme dry heat or a chemical sterilant to remove all microorganisms. Equipment is typically exposed to dry heat during the autoclaving process. Autoclaving is considered to be the most effective method of sterilization. Chemical sterilization is used for equipment unable to tolerate high temperatures, such as fluids and rubber. Care must be taken when handling sterile equipment. Any contact with a non-sterile surface will introduce new microorganisms to the equipment. When a piece of sterile equipment is prepared for use, it should be handled using sterile technique.

## Infection

Infections are divided into two groups, localized and systemic.

1. A localized infection occurs when a virus or bacteria begins to grow in a small area of the body. This can occur in wounds or surgical sites if not treated properly. Signs and symptoms of a localized infection include warmth, redness, and swelling around the site; purulent or foul-smelling drainage; or a fever.
2. In a systemic infection, a virus or bacteria has gained access to the bloodstream, spreading to other parts of the body as a result. Signs of a systemic infection include fever, malaise, nausea, vomiting, chills, and generalized weakness.

### Bacterial and Viral Infection

A bacterial infection is caused when bacteria are introduced into the body. The bacteria multiply to infect the patient, resulting in infection. Bacterial infection is typically localized. For example, a throat infection may result in worse pain on one side of the throat. Antibiotics can be prescribed to help kill bacterial growth.

Viral infections occur when a virus invades through the mucous membranes. It attaches itself to a living cell and uses its genetic material to produce more of the virus. This results in the death of the host cell. Viral infections do not respond to antibiotic treatment. Though some antiviral medications exist, the usual course of treatment in a viral infection is to treat the symptoms and bolster the immune system to fight the infection.

### Microorganism Transmission

Microorganisms must move from one host to another in order to survive.

Some microorganisms are transmitted via droplets that are released when an infected host coughs or sneezes. The microorganisms in the droplets can then invade a new host via the mucous membranes of the eyes, nose, or mouth. Microorganisms may also be transmitted through direct oral contact, such as through kissing an infected person or by drinking from the same cup as the sick individual.

Iatrogenic transmission occurs when microorganisms move to a new host during a medical procedure, such as a surgery or line placement. On rare occasions, microorganisms can be transmitted through the fecal-oral route. This most typically occurs as a result of indirect contact with fecal material, such as through poor hand washing or by eating foods that have been contaminated.

# Personal Care

Activities of daily living (ADLs) are tasks that are required to keep a person healthy and functional. Often, a person's level of health is determined by his ability to perform ADLs. The tasks are divided into two subgroups: basic ADLs and instrumental ADLs.

- Basic ADLs are tasks people must be perform in order to care for themselves. These include bathing, dressing, feeding, toileting, and walking.
- Instrumental ADLs are tasks performed in order to live independently within the community. These include shopping, cooking, housework, medication management, and money management.

**Hygiene**

The components of hygiene are the tasks that are necessary to promote patient health through cleanliness. These tasks include hair care, nail care, mouth care, bathing, and dressing. Hair care includes a gentle brushing and inspection of the patient's scalp. Nail care involves keeping the patient's nails trimmed and inspecting the patient's nail beds. Mouth care is performed to prevent tooth decay and to examine the patient's oral mucosa for sores or signs of infection. Bathing is done to keep the patient's skin clean and to inspect for lesions; this includes perineal care. The nursing aide must also ensure that dependent patients are able to dress and undress themselves properly.

**Bath**

Over time, irritants can build on the patient's skin, which can cause a rash or skin breakdown. These irritants can also cause itching, which may provoke the patient to scratch the skin, creating a source of infection. Bathing cleanses the patient's skin of these irritants. Bathing can also promote patient relaxation and increase circulation. Bathing presents an opportunity to perform a thorough assessment of the patient's skin. Any signs of breakdown or lesions should be immediately reported. Furthermore, the patient's skin should be closely monitored for dryness, as this can cause cracking of the patient's skin.

A tub bath is preferred when the patient is strong enough to get into and out of the bathtub. It involves completely washing the patient, including performing perineal care. A tub bath can be given daily. However, if the patient's skin is showing signs of dryness, the frequency may be reduced to two or three times a week.

A bed bath is given to a patient when he is unable to ambulate. A complete bed bath involves cleansing the patient's skin and changing the patient's linens. If the patient is incontinent of urine or stool, a partial bath may be given. This involves cleansing only those parts of the body that have been soiled and changing only those linens that are dirty.

*Equipment to perform a bed bath:* A bed bath can be a time-consuming procedure, depending upon the patient's level of activity. One way to facilitate a bed bath is to make sure that all of the necessary supplies are present prior to starting the bath.

A nurse aide will require a basin of water, soap, lotion, and baby powder. The water should be warmed to between 105 and 115 degrees. The nurse aide will need several washcloths and at least two towels. The nurse aide should also have a pair of gloves to wear while giving the bath.

Linens should be changed while the bed bath is being performed. In order to change the bed, the nurse aide will need a fitted sheet, a bed pad, a flat sheet, a blanket, and pillowcases.

A.M. and H.S. Care

A.M. care is typically done in the morning, prior to any scheduled medical procedures. A.M. care involves a complete bath, shaving, dressing, hair care, oral care, and nails care, and may require changing of the bed linens.

Hour of sleep (H.S.) care is done at bedtime. H.S. care involves an abbreviated form of skin care, including washing the patient's face and hands. Oral care should also be performed. A back rub may be given for 5 to 10 minutes to ensure the patient is relaxed and ready for sleep. Additional tasks may be performed, depending upon the patient's level of health and activity.

**Hair Care**

Hair care is a procedure that helps to improve patient comfort and morale. It stimulates blood circulation within the scalp. Hair washing also removes excess oils and bacteria. Frequency of hair care depends upon the amount of oil that has accumulated in the patient's hair, as well as the level of dryness of the scalp.

The nurse aide must be vigilant while performing hair care. Head lice, an excessive amount of dandruff, or sores on the scalp should be reported to the nurse immediately if noticed by the nurse aide. Such findings may require special precautions to be taken while performing hair care in the future.

**Patient's Nails**

A nurse aide should exercise caution when providing nail care to patients who are receiving anticoagulation therapy as this type of medication puts the patient at an increased risk for bleeding. Nail care should not be performed on patients with a history of diabetes or decreased circulation in their feet.

Diabetes and low circulation affect the ability of the tissue to repair itself. As a result, even the smallest cut on the skin places the patient at risk for severe ulcers on the feet. Prior to performing nail care; the nurse aide should check the facility policies to ensure that nail cutting falls within her scope of practice.

*Importance of nail care:* Nail care is important for a number of reasons. The primary purpose of nail care is to remove bacteria and dirt from the patient's nail beds, preventing the spread of microorganisms. Appropriate nail care also ensures the patient's nails are not sharp or jagged, which increases the risk of infection from breakage of the skin. While performing nail care, the nursing aide has the opportunity to inspect the patient's nail beds for any signs of inflammation or fungal growth. Any signs of infection or discoloration should immediately be reported to the nurse.

**Four Stages of Pressure Sores**

Pressure sores are divided into four stages, classified by the depth of the wound.

1. Stage I pressure sore refers to an area of redness that is typically located over a bony prominence. The reddened area may feel painful or warm to the touch.
2. Stage II pressure sore refers to wearing away of the first layer of skin, revealing a pink wound bed below.

3. Stage III pressure sore extends past the full thickness of the skin; fatty tissue may be visualized. Tunneling may also be present.
4. Stage IV pressure sore is the most severe, referring to a loss of enough skin tissue to reveal muscle tissue or bone.

## Skin Irritation

Skin irritation can result in sores and infection. There are a number of measures a nurse aide can take to prevent skin irritation from occurring. One way to avoid skin rash or irritation is to completely cleanse the skin of any urine or feces if the patient has soiled himself. Because urine and stool is acidic in nature, skin breakdown can occur quickly if left close to the patient's skin. If the patient is incontinent, applying water resistant lotion will protect the skin by creating a barrier that will prevent rashes or breakdown. Frequent repositioning should also be performed to prevent skin breakdown. A bedridden patient should be turned every two hours to prevent breakdown over bony prominences.

## Oral Care

Performing oral care presents an ideal opportunity to examine the patient's oral mucosa for abnormalities. The nurse aide should carefully observe the patient's mouth for any sores, redness, or bleeding on the patient's lips or gums. Cracking may occur on the patient's lips as a result of dryness. The nurse aide should also be observant for any odor that may occur as a result of infection.

Thrush is a fungal infection that can develop as a result of poor oral care or after taking certain medications. If thrush is present, the patient may appear with white patches covering the tongue or gums. The patient may also complain of a thick, furry feeling in the mouth.

## Dressing a Dependent Patient

When the patient has suffered a stroke, it can result in weakness on one side of the patient's body. Often, the patient may require assistance in daily activities, such as dressing. It is important to teach the patient how to clothe himself safely to promote independence and decrease the risk of falling. Before beginning to assist the patient in undressing, make sure the clean set of clothes is within easy reach. When putting on clothing, the patient should be taught to dress the weakened side first. For example, a patient with weakness on the right side should insert the right arm into the sleeve first. When removing clothes, the patient should be taught to undress the strong side first.

## Measuring Intake and Output

Intake and output (I&O) is an important indicator of fluid balance.

- Intake is calculated by measuring all of the fluid the patient drinks.
- Output is calculated by measuring all of the fluid the patient secretes, including urine, stool, and emesis.

All measurements should be recorded in milliliters (mL). Calculating I&O over a period of a few days can give an indication of the patient's fluid status. Ideally, intake should equal output. If intake exceeds output, then the patient may be fluid overloaded. If output exceeds intake, the patient may be dehydrated.

## Therapeutic Diets

The diet that is prescribed for a patient depends upon the individual's health history.

- A regular diet has no dietary restrictions; patients can eat whatever they like.
- A calorie count diet is typically ordered for diabetic patients; it limits the amount of sugar the patient takes in and counts the number of calories and carbohydrates the patient consumes.
- A low-sodium diet is prescribed to limit the amount of salt ingested by patients with a history of renal impairment or hypertension.
- A cardiac diet is ordered for patients with a history of cardiac problems; while on this diet, they are served low-fat, low-calorie, and low-sodium foods.
- NPO (nothing by mouth) is a diet that is ordered for patients who are not allowed to eat. It is typically ordered in anticipation of medical testing or a surgical procedure. Patient status will also be made NPO if it is unsafe for the individual to eat, such as a patient who is intubated, sedated, or unable to swallow properly.
- A clear liquid diet is the first diet prescribed after a patient is taken off NPO status. It is typically ordered to allow the patient to eat without experiencing nausea.
- A mechanical soft diet is prescribed for patients who have difficulty chewing, such as patients who do not have their dentures. It is also intended to help patients to transition from NPO to a regular diet.

## MyPlate

The USDA's Food Pyramid was heavily criticized for being vague and confusing, and in 2011 it was replaced with MyPlate. MyPlate is much easier to understand, as it consists of a picture of a dinner plate divided into four sections, visually illustrating how our daily diet should be distributed among the various food groups. Vegetables and grains each take up 30% of the plate, while fruits and proteins each constitute 20% of the plate. There is also a representation of a cup, marked Dairy, alongside the plate. The idea behind MyPlate is that it's much easier for people to grasp the idea that half of a meal should consist of fruits and vegetables than it is for them to understand serving sizes for all the different kinds of foods they eat on a regular basis.

*Different types of nutrients and their importance:* Nutrients are elements in nature that are necessary in order to live. Our bodies absorb the nutrients from the foods we eat. Nutrients are divided into six groups: carbohydrates, proteins, fats, minerals, vitamins, and water.

Carbohydrates are composed primarily of sugar and serve as the main source of energy. Protein is made primarily of amino acids and aids in tissue repair. Fats are composed of fatty acids and are essential for cell membrane integrity and thermal regulation. Minerals and vitamins are needed to aid metabolism and a number of other body processes. Water acts as a solvent and is also required for a number of body processes.

*Promotion of hydration:* Water is a vitally important nutrient. It aids in metabolism, temperature regulation, and elimination of body waste. Water is constantly lost through normal sweating, elimination, and exhalation. Certain states, such as illness and increased activity, can cause increased water loss.

It is recommended that the patient take in at least 1500mL to 2000mL or 8 to 10 glasses of water every day to maintain hydration and replace lost body fluids. If the patient does not receive an adequate amount of fluids, dehydration may occur. If left uncorrected, dehydration can be a fatal condition.

## Assist in Feeding

The amount of feeding assistance that should be provided depends upon the individual patient. Some patients will not require assistance to feed themselves. If the patient is able to feed himself, he should be allowed to do so to encourage independence. Some assistance may be required, such as cutting larger portions and opening beverages. Some patients, such as those who suffer from blindness, may only need verbal cues to eat. Some patients are unable to feed themselves as a result of weakness or paralysis of the upper body. These patients will require their food be cut and each bite fed to them. Nurse aides should be careful to take their time and not rush the feeding. Aides should ensure the patient has chewed and swallowed every bite, before offering the next bit of food.

# Mental Health

## Mental Changes Involved in Aging

Cognitive impairment in the elderly typically becomes noticeable at around 60 years of age, though the rate of decline varies depending on the individual. As a person ages, he typically experiences a mild decline in the ability to retrieve words and name common objects. Memory also tends to decline as a person ages. The ability to encode new information declines, typically as a result of a decline in sensory abilities. Short-term memory may also decline, though significant changes in long-term memory are typically not seen until about 70 to 80 years of age. The rate of memory decline can be stemmed using memory exercises and problem-solving skills.

## Agitated Patient

When a patient becomes agitated, the key is to remain calm. Remind the patient who you are, and attempt to reorient the patient to the surroundings. Speak calmly and clearly; attempt to learn what it is that is causing the patient to become agitated. Treat the patient as you want him to behave. While talking to the patient, assume a non-threatening posture. If possible, enlist the aid of family members to calm the patient down. If all of these measures fail and the patient is behaving in a way that may cause harm to himself or to other people, restraints may be required.

## Confused Patient

Confusion that develops in the hospital or extended-care facility is typically a symptom of a physiological problem. If the nurse aide notices confusion in a patient who was previously oriented, the nurse should be notified immediately.

The nurse aide should try to find out what the patient's normal orientation was prior to entering the hospital; this can be done by reviewing records and talking to family members. The nurse aide should be observant for any signs of the physiological problem that may be causing the confusion. For example, cloudy urine may indicate a urinary tract infection, which could result in confusion in the elderly. Until the cause of the confusion is determined, the nurse aide should provide a safe, non-threatening environment while attempting to reorient the patient to the surroundings.

## Reality Orientation

Reality orientation is a set of activities that are performed with a confused patient in an attempt to reorient him to his environment. The first step of reality orientation is to approach the patient in a friendly, non-threatening manner. While interacting with the patient, the nurse aide should provide verbal reminders regarding time and place. The nurse aide should provide the patient with physical reminders of the surroundings, such as writing the date on a whiteboard within the patient's visual field or showing the patient where a clock can be located.

## Depression

Depression is a disorder in which the patient experiences a consistently low mood, coupled with feelings of worthlessness, sadness, or self-loathing. The patient may experience insomnia (inability to sleep) or hypersomnia (sleeping too much). The patient may also complain of digestive difficulties or frequent headaches. Severe cases of depression may result in increased forgetfulness or hallucinations.

Depression can be caused by a number of physical, psychological, or sociological factors. Physical characteristics, such as a small hippocampus of the brain, may lead to the onset of depression. Depression may also be brought on by life-altering illnesses, such as Parkinson's disease, heart attack, or stroke. Tragic life events and the inability to effectively cope with them may also lead to an onset of depression.

# Care Impaired

## Patient Orientation

There a number of methods that a nursing aide can use to orient a patient to a new facility. If the patient is only there for a short stay, it may only be necessary to orient him to his room. This includes orienting the patient to the bed controls; call light, and any continuous equipment he may be using, such as telemetry equipment or pulse oximetry. The patient should also be given any necessary information regarding unit policies and visiting hours. If the patient is expected to stay for a long period of time, such as at an extended-care facility, he should also be given a brief tour of the unit. If the facility allows it, the patient may benefit from being introduced to other ambulatory patients.

## Alzheimer's Disease

Alzheimer's disease is a degenerative disorder of the brain. It is the most common cause of dementia. It typically affects people 65 years of age and older, though early onset Alzheimer's disease can occur. The cause of Alzheimer's disease is unknown. Initial symptoms of Alzheimer's disease include loss of short-term memory or forgetfulness. As the disease progresses the patient experiences increasing confusion and aggression, while losing long-term memory, language skills, and other cognitive functions. Death typically results from breakdown of bodily functions. Alzheimer's disease is incurable; management of the disease is the key to an extended life expectancy after diagnosis.

## Parkinson's Disease

Parkinson's disease is a disorder that results in degeneration of the nervous system. It causes a decline in speech and motor skills and may cause a decline in cognitive function. Typical signs of Parkinson's disease include tremulousness, a shuffling gait, difficulty turning, difficulty speaking or swallowing, and a mask-like face. Parkinson's disease may also result in short-term memory loss and dementia in advanced cases. In most cases, the cause of Parkinson's disease is unknown, though in some cases the cause may be genetic or a result of a history of head trauma. Treatment includes medication management, management of symptoms, and surgery.

## Dementia

Dementia is a term used to describe any cognitive dysfunction that may occur as a result of long-term illness, such as Alzheimer's disease, depression, and cerebral vascular accident.

Dementia encompasses any resulting difficulties in memory, language, or problem-solving abilities. The patient is usually considered to be demented after six months of cognitive dysfunction; cognitive dysfunction that has gone on less than six months is typically referred to as delirium. Dementia may be curable, depending upon the cause. If the patient starts showing any signs of confusion, it should be reported to the nurse immediately.

### Irreversible Dementia

Multi-infarct dementia is the second most common cause of irreversible cognitive dysfunction. It is caused by tissue damage that occurs when atherosclerotic plaque on the vessel wall breaks off and migrates to another part of the brain, where it creates a blockage. Because the brain tissue cannot get an adequate supply of blood flow, brain tissue in the area of the blockage dies from hypoxia. Though the blockages can be treated, cognitive function does not return after treatment.

Huntington's disease is the degeneration of certain types of brain cells. Dementia often develops in the late stages of this disease.

<u>Common Causes</u>

There are a number of diseases and disorders that result in the onset of dementia. The most common cause of dementia is infection of the brain, such as meningitis or encephalitis. Both the infection and the resulting dementia typically resolve after treatment with antibiotics.

Disorders that cause undue pressure on the brain, such as head injuries, hydrocephalus, and brain tumors, can cause dementia. There are treatments available to treat the increased pressure, and the dementia diminishes after the pressure has been relieved. Disorders that affect other body systems, such as liver disease, kidney disease, or pancreatic disease, can cause dementia by upsetting the delicate chemical balance within the body. In order to restore the patient's previous mental state, the chemical balance in the body must be restored.

## Sundowner's Syndrome

Sundowner's syndrome is a condition in which patients become increasingly confused in the late afternoon or early evening. It is most commonly seen in patients with a history of Alzheimer's disease or dementia; however, it can occur in patients who do not have a history of dementia. Though a number of theories exist as to why Sundowner's syndrome occurs, the actual cause is unknown. Patients who are suffering from Sundowner's syndrome may experience worsening confusion, restlessness, or agitation. Some patients may experience hallucinations or wandering as part of Sundowner's syndrome.

*Steps a nurse aide can take to alleviate the symptoms of Sundowner's syndrome:* There are a number of steps a nurse aide can take to decrease the severity of Sundowner's syndrome.

- In the morning, the nurse aide should open the curtains and blinds and allow the patient to see outside to reorient them to time of day.
- Encourage exercise during the day.
- Plan all strenuous activities for the morning so that there is an adequate amount of time to relax prior to bedtime.
- Do not allow the patient to sleep during the day as this will make it difficult to sleep during the night.
- Plan a few relaxing activities before bed, such as therapeutic massage or quiet reading time.
- These activities should be performed at the same time every night to establish a routine.
- When it is time to sleep, darken the room as much as possible to further reinforce time of day.

## Visual Impairment Patient

A nurse aide should take special precautions when caring for a patient who has a visual impairment. Prior to interacting with the patient, the nurse aide should acquaint herself with the type of visual impairment the patient has. She should make sure to identify herself as soon as she enters the room and stand within the patient's visual field while interacting with him. While ambulating the patient, the nurse aide should allow the patient to move as freely as possible and provide clear verbal cues regarding potential obstacles. The furniture in the patient's room should not be moved to allow the patient to become familiar with the surroundings.

## Hearing Impaired Patient

If the patient has difficulty hearing in one ear the nurse aide should talk while standing on the side that the patient can hear. The nurse aide should introduce herself and speak slowly and clearly. The nurse aide should face the patient while talking to give him the opportunity to read lips. While talking to the patient, the nurse aide should try to limit background noise and deepen the tone of her voice in order to make herself heard. If the patient can see well, communication can be achieved using written messages rather than speaking.

## Aphasia

Aphasia is defined as difficulty speaking that result from lesions on the brain. Aphasia is typically caused by cerebral vascular accident, brain injury, brain tumors, or by progressive diseases, such as Alzheimer's disease or Parkinson's disease. Aphasia can come in a number of different forms.

- The patient may be unable to speak or may speak using inappropriate words and phrases.
- The patient may become unable to name objects or call objects by the wrong names.
- Aphasia can also affect the patient's ability to comprehend language.
- With aphasia, the patient may become unable to read, write, or form complete sentences.

*Caring for a patient with aphasia:* Prior to interacting with the patient, the nurse aide should acquaint herself with the type of aphasia the patient has and communicate with the patient accordingly.

The key to caring for a patient with aphasia is to avoid becoming frustrated. Do not rush the patient; allow him time to gather his thoughts and say what he is trying to say. Avoid attempting to speak for the patient. Try to use a picture or letter board to assist with communication. If possible, allow the patient to write messages in order to communicate.

# Resident Rights

## Patient's Bill of Rights

The Patient's Bill of Rights is a list of rights that the patient can expect to receive while he stays in a hospital or an extended-care facility. This list of rights may differ in wording from hospital to hospital but generally contains similar provisions.

- The Bill of Rights is typically accompanied by a list of responsibilities that the patient should adhere to in order to ensure his treatment is effective.
- It is important that the patient be made aware of his rights and responsibilities as soon after admission as possible.

## HIPAA Act

Congress enacted the Health Insurance Portability and Accountability Act (HIPAA) in 1996 in order to ensure the privacy of patient health information. It requires each health care facility to prepare a list of policies and procedures in order to protect patient information. This includes limiting the ability to access patient information to only those who provide direct patient care.

HIPAA also requires each health care facility to come up with technological safeguards to prevent the removal of patient information from hospital computer systems. If the hospital system violates the standards set forth by HIPAA, the hospital may be subject to severe fines and other penalties.

## Right of Privacy

Patients have a right to personal privacy. The nursing aide should make an effort to protect the patient's privacy by maintaining his dignity during patient care procedures. While bathing the patient or taking him off of the bedpan, the curtain or door to the room should be closed to prevent other people from seeing in.

The patient's right to privacy also applies to his health information. Details of the patient's case should only be discussed with the family members that the patient specifies. Many facilities have developed a system involving a privacy code number that is only given to the family members that are to receive information regarding the patient. Unless the family member is able to provide the privacy code number, the nursing aide can only confirm the patient's presence on the unit.

## Right of Confidentiality

The patient has the right to have his case discussed only by those who are directly responsible for his care. Unless a nursing aide is caring for the patient, she should not review his chart or discuss his case. Furthermore, once the nursing aide is no longer providing care to the patient, she should not access his records.

After the patient is transferred to another unit of the hospital, the nursing aide should not access his files. Patient information should be discussed in areas where other people cannot overhear it to prevent laypeople from hearing details about the patient's care.

## Right of Respectful Care

When a patient enters the hospital, he has the right to be treated respectfully by those who are providing care to him. The patient cannot be discriminated against because of age, gender, race, or religion.

He also cannot be denied treatment as a result of the circumstances surrounding his hospitalization. For example, the patient cannot be denied care for injuries acquired during the commission of a crime. While the patient is in the hospital, he has the right to expect care to be provided safely by competent staff. While the patient is in the hospital or extended-care facility, reasonable measures should be taken to accommodate the patient's cultural or religious requests, provided they do not interfere with the care of other patients.

## Right of Informed Consent

The idea of informed consent originally came about in reference to experimental treatment. However, it has come to encompass the type of information that should be provided prior to every test, procedure, or treatment.

Before signing the consent form, the patient has the right to be informed about all of the risks and benefits involved in the proposed treatment, as well as the risks and benefits involved in refusing the treatment. He should be told which doctors will be involved in his care and what medications he will receive. The doctor should provide this information prior to the procedure, either directly to the patient or to the patient's health care power of attorney.

## Right of Freedom of Choice

The patient's right to freedom of choice works in conjunction with the right of informed consent. Once he has been provided the necessary information, the patient has the right to choose what treatments he will receive. He is free to make this decision without pressure from the health care staff. Once he has made his decision, it cannot be undermined unless he makes the decision to change treatments. Conversely, if the patient decides to stop the treatment, he may do so, though the doctor should remind the patient about the risks and benefits involved in quitting the treatment.

## Patient's Telephone and Mail Rights

The patient has the right to have regular access to a telephone in order to communicate with family members. The patient should be informed as to where the telephone is located and how to use it. The patient should also have an expectation of privacy during his telephone conversations. The patient's conversations should not be monitored or recorded in any way.

The patient has similar rights regarding the mail. Patient mail should not be opened without his consent, and any outgoing mail should be sent without being read by members of the health care staff.

## Patient Rights to See Their Chart

If the patient demands to see his chart, the nursing aide should notify the charge nurse. Though it is the patient's right to see his chart, most facilities have a policy regarding patient chart review. Such a request is typically forwarded to the medical records department, who will make copies of the patient's chart to provide to the patient. This prevents the patient from potentially altering the information in his chart. Copies of the chart are typically provided within 10 days of the initial request. There may be forms for the patient to fill out prior to receiving copies of his chart, and the charge nurse or someone from the medical records department will provide the forms for him.

## DNR Order

A Do Not Resuscitate order outlines the type of heroic measures that may be undertaken if the patient's heart or breathing were to stop during the course of treatment. The DNR order typically specifies if the patient desires emergent intubation, CPR, or defibrillation. The doctor typically writes a DNR order after an extensive conversation with the patient about his wishes regarding his care.

In some cases, the patient may choose to have some of the emergency treatments, but not all of them. It is important for the nursing aide to familiarize herself with the types of emergency treatment the patient wants. The patient can reverse a DNR at any time. If the patient verbalizes a desire to change his code status, the charge nurse should be notified.

## Advanced Directives

Advanced directives detail the patient's wishes regarding end-of-life care. They address whether the patient wants to receive long-term mechanical ventilation, continuous dialysis, or nourishment via a feeding tube. The advanced directives may also address whether the patient wants to be an organ or tissue donor after death. The patient typically sees a lawyer to have his advanced directives prepared prior to hospitalization. Health care providers should be made aware immediately upon hospitalization if the patient has advanced directives. If the patient's family brings in a copy of the patient's advanced directives, the nursing aide should notify the nurse immediately.

## Medical Durable Power of Attorney

A medical durable power of attorney designates a specific person to make any medically related decisions if the patient should become unable to make the decisions himself. Durable power of attorney would take effect if the patient were to become confused or comatose. The durable power of attorney is typically filed by a lawyer prior to hospitalization. The person who has been made medical power of attorney should make an effort to learn the patient's wishes regarding health care decisions. If the patient becomes hospitalized, the family should present the durable power of attorney paperwork as soon as possible. If the patient's family brings in a copy of the patient's durable power of attorney, the nursing aide should inform the nurse immediately.

## Right to Continuity of Care

Continuity of care is defined as high-quality health care provided continuously and consistently. Often, continuity of care can be difficult to achieve in a health care setting because of the number of practitioners that can get involved in a patient's case. Continuity of care may break down for a number of reasons, including a doctor's lack of familiarity with a treatment plan or lack of communication among the health care team. In order to maintain continuity of care, there should be frequent conferences between the health care team and the patient to ensure that everyone is in agreement regarding the plan of care.

## Patient's Experimental Treatment

The patient has very specific rights when it comes to experimental treatment. Like any other procedure, informed consent is required prior to beginning treatment.

- The patient should be notified of the experimental nature of the treatment, as well as any potential risks and benefits involved in accepting the treatment.
- The patient should be approached in a manner that is not threatening.
- If the patient refuses the treatment, he has the right to be informed of other treatments that may be performed in place of the experimental treatment.
- Care cannot be refused to the patient based upon refusal of an experimental treatment.

## Patient's Right of Refusal

If the patient is alert and oriented, he has the right to refuse any treatment or procedure. This includes simple procedures, such as turning or a bath. If the patient decides, for example, that he does not want to be turned, he should not be scolded or coerced for his decision. He should be informed of the risks involved in not being turned. If the patient continues to refuse, then the nursing aide should not argue. The charge nurse should be notified so that the proper documentation can be made. If possible, the nursing aide may offer the procedure again at a later time.

## Leaving the Health Care Facility

As long as the patient is alert and oriented, he may choose to leave the health care facility at any time. If the patient states a desire to leave, the nursing aide should inform the charge nurse immediately. The charge nurse will talk to the patient and attempt to discover the reason that he wants to leave. If the patient cannot be convinced to stay and is considered competent to make that decision, the doctor will be notified of the patient's decision. In many cases, the patient will be asked to sign an AMA form, indicating that he acknowledges that he is leaving Against Medical Advice. It is not the responsibility of the nursing aide to obtain the patient's signature.

## Identification of Health Care Workers

The patient has the right to know the names of the people that are providing care for him. On a given day, the patient may encounter a number of people, including doctors, nurses, physical therapists, and nursing aides. A name badge clearly identifies a person as an employee of the health care facility and states the individual's position. It informs the patient of what to expect from the employee. When a nursing aide enters the patient's room, she should wear her nametag above the waist in a location that is clearly visible. She should also identify herself in order to prevent confusion.

## Money and Valuables

Though it is unwise to bring a large sum of money or valuables to a hospital setting, it is sometimes unavoidable. Dentures and hearing aids, for example, are very costly pieces of equipment, but they are also necessary for everyday use.

If the patient enters the hospital with money or valuables, he has the right to expect that the hospital will take reasonable steps to protect his property. The patient has the right to maintain his own accounts when he enters a long-term care facility. At no point should a member of the health care facility access the patient's financial accounts. If the patient is unable to take responsibility for his financial matters, the social worker should be contacted to make necessary arrangements.

## Protect Patient Valuables

If the patient comes into the hospital with large sums of money or jewelry, the patient should be encouraged to give it to a family member to take home. If a family member is not present, permission should be obtained from the patient to put the valuables in the hospital safe. If the patient consents, security should be called, the items catalogued, and a receipt given to the patient. If the patient is unconscious or comatose, the valuables should be locked up until he is able to give consent. If the patient has a valuable that is required for daily use, such as glasses, hearing aids, or dentures, every effort must be taken to protect these items. The patient should be provided a case marked with his name on it. When the items are not in use, they should be kept close at hand in a place where they are not at risk for breaking or being lost.

## Dying Patient Rights

A patient's rights should be closely respected at all times, especially when he is dying. Every effort should be made to place the patient in a private room. When the family is present, the door to the room should be closed; if the door cannot be closed, then the curtain should be pulled shut. Reports regarding the patient should be given where others cannot overhear. Any monitor alarms should be turned off or silenced. Privacy should be respected if the patient needs to be cleaned up and during postmortem care. When transporting the body to the morgue, the morgue cart should be kept covered to protect the patient's identity.

## Culture

Culture is defined as the behavior and belief systems of a particular group. A person's cultural outlook is shaped by ethnicity, gender, and age. It affects his outlook on all things, including health care.

It can affect the types of foods the patient might eat while sick, his behaviors during illness, and his attitude about death and dying. The patient's cultural beliefs should be taken into account when planning care. If the patient's cultural beliefs are not taken into account, it may increase the patient's stress level, hindering the healing process.

## Religion

Religion is the set of beliefs that the person has regarding the nature of the universe. The patient's religion may dictate the level of participation in his care, including what treatments he may accept. Religion can also aid in the patient's ability to cope during the recovery period following serious illness or injury. The patient's religious outlook should be taken into account when planning the patient's care. Failure to do so may result in the patient's refusal to participate in the care or withdrawal from the hospital setting altogether.

## Patient's Special Dietary Needs

Upon admission to the hospital or long-term care facility the nurse aide should make note of any cultural or religious requests that the patient may have regarding dietary needs. The facility dietary service should be notified as soon as possible to ensure the patient is provided with appropriate foods. Prior to taking the tray in to the room, the nurse aide should check to make sure the food on the tray meet the patient's dietary restrictions. If it does not, the dietary service should be notified regarding the problem, and a replacement meal should be obtained as soon as possible.

## Patient Asks to See a Priest

During times of illness or injury, it is not uncommon for a patient to request to see a priest or a person of authority within his church. If a patient makes such a request the nurse aide should notify the charge nurse immediately. The charge nurse will talk with the patient and find out if there is a specific person the patient wishes to see. Most hospitals and extended-care facilities have an on-call clergyperson who can be notified if the patient does not have a specific person to call.

## Christian Patient

It is important for the nursing aide to ask if the patient has any dietary restrictions. Though most Christians do not have dietary restrictions as a result of their faith, some may have self-imposed dietary restrictions.

Some Catholic patients may wish to fast during Lent. During their stay, some Catholic or Orthodox Christian patients may choose to receive communion or give confession during their hospitalization.

Some patients may request to receive Last Rites if they are critically ill or dying. It is important to notify the charge nurse immediately if the patient requests to see a priest during his stay. In many cases, the patient or family will know a priest they would want to call.

## Muslim Patient

It is important to ask the patient if he has any specific dietary restrictions. Many strict practicing Muslims will eat only specially slaughtered fish, chicken, and beef. Most Muslims will not eat pork products.

Try to avoid handing a Muslim patient anything with the left hand as that is the hand that is reserved for performing perineal care on oneself. Muslims place a strong emphasis on cleanliness. Many Muslims prefer to wash with soap and water after using the bedpan, rather than using toilet paper. They should also be provided with fresh water to wash with prior to their prayers.

If possible, female patients should be cared for by female nursing aides.

## Jewish Patient

Orthodox Jews eat only kosher meat and typically avoid dishes in which milk and meat have been prepared together.

Other types of foods that are forbidden include pork products, meat from birds of prey, and shellfish.

Most Jewish patients prefer to wash their hands and say a brief prayer prior to eating; the nursing aide should provide them with an opportunity to do so. Jewish men may prefer to remain bearded or may choose to shave using an electric razor rather than a razor blade.

Jewish patients observe specific practices regarding death. The family will notify their Synagogue of the patient's impending death; if there is no family present, the health care staff should do so. After the death, three members of the family typically wash the body. Burial should take place within 24 hours after dying.

## Hindu Patient

It is important for the nursing aide to inquire about any specific dietary needs. Most Hindus are vegetarian or vegan; even those that do eat meat may refuse to eat beef or pork.

After using the bedpan, most Hindu patients prefer to wash their perineal area using clean water rather than using toilet paper. The nursing aide should make it available if requested.

Some Hindus may prefer to wash in the shower rather than sitting in the bath. Members of the Hindu faith particularly value privacy; if possible, the patient should be cared for by a nursing aide who is of the same gender.

Some Hindu patients may prefer to die while lying on the ground to maintain closeness between the individual and Mother Earth. If necessary, a Hindu priest may be called in to perform holy rites for the patient.

## Buddhist Patient

It is important for a nursing aide to inquire about a Buddhist's dietary needs on admission as many Buddhist patients are vegetarians or vegans.

Many Buddhists fast on specific days, including the days of the New Moon and Full Moon. On fasting days, a Buddhist will only eat at specific times. The nursing aide should collaborate with the patient on these days to ensure he gets his meal tray at appropriate times.

The type of rituals surrounding death and dying varies depending on the patient's traditions. The patient may request a Buddhist monk or nun to perform chants in order to assist in the patient's passing. If possible, the body should not be touched until 3 to 8 hours after death before preparing the body for death.

## Mormon Patient

Many Mormons follow a set of dietary restrictions put forward in the Word of Wisdom. It teaches against the use of stimulants, such as coffee, tea, and other caffeinated beverages. Though most Mormons are not strict vegetarians, they do tend to eat meat sparingly.

Some Mormons may wear a special undergarment that should be treated with the utmost privacy. It can be removed for laundering and washing but is otherwise worn at all times.

Though Mormons do not have specific rites or rituals regarding a dying patient, the nursing aide should make sure to allow the family to spend as much time as possible with the patient in his final hours. If the patient wears the sacred undergarment, it should be put back on the body after postmortem care has been performed.

## Patients with Disabilities

Every effort should be taken to protect the rights of patients with disabilities.

- If the patient is hearing or visually impaired, the health care team should tailor its communication techniques to make sure the patient understands what is being said to him.
- If the patient is confused or mentally challenged, the patient's health care proxy must be kept informed of his status and conferred with regarding aspects of his care.
- If the patient does not have a health care proxy and there is no family available, a temporary proxy can be named to act in the patient's best interests until the patient is well enough to do so himself.
- If necessary, the health care facility's social work team should be notified to aid in protecting the rights of a patient with disabilities.

# Communication

## Therapeutic Communication

Therapeutic communication is a method of communicating with patients that encourages them to open up and provide information. Because of the level of stress involved in hospitalization, the patient often needs to communicate but is unsure how to initiate conversation with the health care staff.

Therapeutic communication combines a variety of verbal and nonverbal communication techniques in order to encourage the patient to speak openly. By making note of the patient's body language as well as his words, the nurse aide can interpret the patient's emotional state and communicate with the patient effectively.

## Communication Components

There are five components that must be present in order for communication to take place.

1.  The first component is the sender. The sender is the original source of the message.
2.  The next component is the message itself or what the sender is trying to convey.
3.  Another component of communication is the channel or the means through which the message is being conveyed. This is typically done using either verbal or nonverbal communication.
4.  The fourth component is the receiver or the person who is receiving the message.
5.  The final component is feedback or the response to the original message. The role of the sender and the receiver may interchange during the course of a conversation.

## Verbal Communication

Verbal communication is one way in which people communicate. It encompasses what is said as well as the way it is said. When communicating with the patient, the nurse aide should take into account the patient's language and word choice, as well as the tone of voice and the volume at which the words are spoken. When talking with a patient, it is important to think carefully about what you say before you say it as words can often be misunderstood. It is also important to ensure that your comments are appropriate to the setting and conversation.

## Nonverbal Communication

Nonverbal communication is the process of sending messages using methods other than speaking. It can convey emotions and attitudes and can aid in communicating effectively with the patient. A person can communicate nonverbally using gestures, touch, or body language.

A nurse aide should closely monitor her own body language to make sure that it does not contradict what she is saying. For example, a nurse aide who talks to the patient while frequently checking her watch is indicating that she is in a hurry. Such body language discourages open communication and should be avoided.

## Encourage Communication

There are a number of steps the nursing aide can take in order to encourage communication with the patient. First, the nurse aide can ensure the patient is in an environment in which he can communicate freely. If the patient is comfortable, he is more likely to participate in therapeutic

- 48 -

conversation. The nurse aide should also ensure the patient's privacy during the conversation. The patient may feel embarrassed about sharing personal information in a public setting. The nursing aide should make an effort to appear unhurried, encouraging the patient to talk by sitting near the patient during the conversation. The nursing aide should also convey interest by facing the patient and maintaining eye contact during the conversation.

## Talking to a Patient Effectively

When the nursing aide is talking to the patient, there are a number of ways she can make sure that what she is saying is clearly communicated.

- The nursing aide should avoid using medical terminology while talking to the patient as many find it to be confusing.
- The nursing aide should make an effort to use words that can be understood by the layman. For example, instead of saying 'hypertension', the nursing aide can be better understood by using the phrase 'high blood pressure'.
- If a medical term must be used, the nursing aide should define the term for the patient.
- While talking with the patient, the nursing aide should speak slowly and clearly in a moderate tone of voice.

## Silence

Silence can be an effective communication tool because it can convey a number of emotions. While communicating with the patient, silence can convey the sentiment of affection. This type of silence is typically accompanied by nonverbal actions, such as a hug or holding the patient's hand. Silence can also be utilized to encourage the patient to give more information. If this is done during a conversation, the patient may continue to talk to fill the silence. Silence can also give the patient time for contemplation. Care must be taken in utilizing silence as a communication tool as it can sometimes be misinterpreted as hostility or rudeness.

## Active Listening

Active listening is the method of listening attentively to the conversation at hand. During a typical conversation, it is not uncommon for a person to not devote her full attention to what is being said. She may be thinking of other things or focusing on the work she is trying to do. When a person is listening actively, she is not only paying attention to the conversation, but also considering the patient's words and forming an appropriate response that will encourage further conversation. Active listening also takes into account various aspects of nonverbal communication in order to draw the appropriate conclusions from the conversation.

## Encouraging Communication

Asking questions can be effective in encouraging communication with the patient. There are two types of questions, open-ended and closed-ended. Open-ended questions encourage the patient to provide added detail about the subject of the conversation, while giving him more control over the conversation. "How do you feel about that?" is an example of an open-ended question. Closed-ended questions can be used to focus the conversation or get it back on track. They are typically used to elicit a short answer. An example of a closed-ended question is "What would you like for lunch?"

## Therapeutic Communication

A general lead is a device used to encourage the patient to continue speaking about a particular subject. Examples of general leads include phrases such as 'go on' or 'I see.' These are effective because they allow the patient to guide the conversation, giving him the opportunity to voice his thoughts and concerns. General leads also indicate that the nurse aide is paying attention to what is being said. When a nursing aide restates something, she rephrases a comment that the patient made earlier in the conversation in order to encourage the patient to elaborate on it. For example, the nursing aide might say, "So you think you have too much equipment on you?" if the patient makes a comment about all of the tubes and wires attached to him.

## Reflecting

Reflecting is another method of encouraging the patient to talk about a particular subject. A nursing aide reflects a statement by repeating all or part of the patient's original statement back to the patient. For example, the patient says, "I feel so lonely." An appropriate reflective response would be "Lonely?" Another form of reflecting is to make a statement regarding the patient's feelings. For example, the nursing aide may say, "It seems like you are very happy about this." This reflects the patient's emotional state and encourages him to speak openly about what he is thinking and feeling.

## Providing Information and Self-Disclosing

Providing information can be an effective tool in encouraging communication. When the patient is new to the health care facility, he may feel anxious about the unfamiliar surroundings. The nursing aide can help ease anxiety by providing the patient with information that is relevant to his care. However, the nurse aide must be careful not to provide specific information regarding the patient's diagnosis or test and lab results.

A nursing aide can also encourage communication by providing some information about herself in order to ease the patient's discomfort. However, the nursing aide must be careful not to dominate the conversation as the goal of therapeutic communication is to discover what the patient is thinking and feeling.

## Touch and Empathy

Empathy is the ability to understand what the patient is feeling and to respond appropriately. Acting empathically begins by recognizing any strong emotions the patient might be having. By recognizing these emotions the nursing aide can give the patient the opportunity to talk about his feelings, as well as provide validation. Acting empathically allows the nursing aide to build trust and understanding with the patient. Using touch is a nonverbal method of communicating with the patient. There are times when words are not enough to provide an adequate amount of comfort. In these times, holding a hand or giving a hug can do more to encourage conversation and provide comfort.

## Communication Block

A communication block is a statement or behavior that discourages therapeutic communication. A nursing aide may inadvertently use a communication block if she is hurried or is uncomfortable about the conversation at hand. Common communication blocks include the use of sarcasm or jokes in order to deflect the situation. The nursing aide may change the subject or may attempt to minimize the problem in order to ease her own discomfort. Offering false assurances or telling the patient how he should feel in a given situation may discourage the patient from communicating with the nursing aide.

## Call Light

The call light is the way in which a patient notifies the health care staff that he is in need of assistance. It should be answered promptly and courteously. If a call light is going off in a room that is not assigned to you, it is appropriate to answer it to find out what the patient needs. When using an intercom the nurse aide should answer by asking, "May I help you?" If answering the call light personally, the nurse aide should introduce herself and inquire about the patient's needs. It is not appropriate for the nursing aide to ignore a call light if she is busy.

### Patient Continual Use of Call Light

Frequent use of the call bell can occur for a number of reasons. The patient may not understand how to use the call bell or may push the wrong button accidentally. If this happens, a nurse aide can tape a piece of gauze over the button so that the patient can recognize the call button using his fingers. If using this method, it is important to check to make sure the call button can be pushed easily prior to leaving the room.

Another reason that a patient may call frequently is that he is lonely. If this is the case, the nurse aide should make an effort to stop in to see the patient as frequently as possible. This may prevent frequent calls 'just to chat. One way to prevent frequent use of the call bell is to make sure the patient has all necessary items within reach prior to leaving the room. Also, ask the patient if there is anything else he might need prior to leaving the room.

## If You Do Not Know How to Perform a Procedure

Nursing aides must perform a variety of tasks while caring for a patient. Some tasks may be performed on a daily basis, while other tasks may be rarely done. If a nursing aide is assigned a task that she does not know how to do she should talk privately with the charge nurse after the assignment has been made to acquire instructions on how to perform the task. If there is still a question about how to perform the task, the nursing aide should check the facility's policies and procedures manual. It typically contains an overview of how to perform a number of common procedures.

## Patient's Inappropriate Comments

Some patients may attempt to use sexual innuendo jokingly or as a way to ease their own discomfort. However, such comments are considered to be harassment. Members of the health care staff have a right to work in an environment that is free of harassment. Some may try to diffuse the situation with a joke, but this approach is typically ineffective in halting the abusive behavior.

If the patient begins making inappropriate comments, the nurse aide should immediately inform the patient that his comments are unacceptable and will not be tolerated. This should be stated firmly, but politely. If the patient continues the inappropriate behavior, the charge nurse should be notified.

## Non-English Speaking Patient

Patients who are unable to speak English may be a challenge to communicate with. Though it is possible to ask a family member to aide in translating, many facilities prefer to use an official interpreter when conveying medically related information to the patient. Whether communicating through a family member or an interpreter, the nursing aide should look at the patient and address him while speaking. She should speak slowly and clearly, and watch the patient's body language and facial expressions closely as this can aide in the communication process. Before the family leaves, the nurse aide should ask them to write down a few common phrases, such as 'bathroom' and 'water,' to help with meeting the patient's needs.

## Communicating with the Patient's Family

Interaction with the patient's family can occur frequently during the course of patient care. The nurse aide can confer with the patient's family regarding procedures that are part of the nursing aide's scope of practice. When talking with the family while the patient is in the room, the nursing aide should make an effort to include the patient in the conversation; it is inappropriate to talk about the patient as if he is not there.

The nursing aide cannot impart information about the patient's prognosis nor can she give information about test or lab results. If a family member has a question about the patient's care, he should be referred to the charge nurse.

### Unable to Communicate with the Patient

Sometimes the nursing aide may be unable to communicate with the patient despite her best efforts. If the patient is intubated or has severe aphasia, he may not be able to effectively communicate his needs. The nursing aide should attempt to figure out what the patient is trying to say by running through a list of common needs, such as being thirsty, hot, cold, or in pain. If the nursing aide cannot figure out what the patient is trying to say, she should tell the patient that she is unable to understand him. She should not pretend to understand as this behavior can cause distress for the patient.

The inability to communicate often results in frustration on the part of the patient. If this happens, the nursing aide should provide appropriate reassurance and emotional support.

# Data Collection

## Collecting a Clean-Catch Urine Specimen

Care must be taken while collecting a urine specimen to make sure that it does not become contaminated during the collection process.

- A clean-catch urine specimen can be collected from a patient who is able to void.
- Provide the patient with a sterile specimen cup.
- Instruct the patient to wash his hands and perineal area thoroughly prior to voiding.
- The patient should start the stream of urine and urinate for at least 2 seconds before beginning to collect urine in the cup.
- Don a pair of gloves.
- Once the patient has acquired a suitable specimen, close the specimen cup tightly and place it in a lab specimen bag.
- Encourage the patient to wash his hands.
- Remove the gloves, and wash your hands.

### Urine Specimen from a Foley Catheter

When collecting a urine specimen from a catheter bag, care must be taken to ensure germs are not introduced into the Foley tubing as this may cause a urinary tract infection.

- Wash your hands, don a pair of gloves, and explain to the patient what you are going to do.
- Clamp the catheter tubing 6 inches above the drainage bag, and allow urine to collect in the tubing.
- Thoroughly clean the collection hub with an alcohol swab.
- Carefully access the collection hub using a Luer-Lok syringe.
- Collect the desired amount of urine.
- Transfer the urine from the syringe into the specimen cup, taking care not to touch the cup with the syringe.
- Tightly close the lid of the specimen cup, and place it in a lab specimen bag.
- Unclamp the catheter tubing.
- Dispose of the syringe.
- Remove the gloves, and wash your hands.

## Collecting a Sputum Specimen

A sputum specimen is often collected to check for infections in the patient's respiratory tract. To collect a sputum specimen:

- Wash your hands, put on a pair of gloves, and explain to the patient what you are going to do.
- Encourage the patient to cough forcefully to expel sputum from the upper respiratory tract.
- Instruct the patient to spit the sputum specimen into the cup.
- If the secretions are thin and clear, it may simply be saliva from the mouth; this is not an adequate specimen.
- Close the lid of the specimen cup tightly, and place it into a lab specimen bag.
- Remove the gloves, and wash your hands.

## Collecting a Stool Specimen

A stool specimen is collected from the patient if there is suspicion of an infection or bleeding in the bowels. When the patient needs to move his bowels:

- Wash your hands, don a pair of gloves, and explain to the patient what you are going to do.
- Position a hat in the commode to catch stool without catching urine as well.
- Assist the patient to the bedside commode, provide privacy, and allow him to move his bowels.
- After assisting the patient back to bed, place a small amount of stool into a sterile specimen cup and close the lid tightly.
- Place the specimen cup into a lab collection bag.
- Dispose of the remaining stool and the hat.
- Remove your gloves, and wash your hands.

## Sterile Gloves

Sterile gloves must be put on carefully to ensure germs are not introduced onto the sterile surface.

- Wash your hands, and dry them thoroughly.
- Unfold the package of gloves, and lay it on a flat surface.
- Using your nondominant hand, grasp the glove intended for your dominant hand at the fold of the cuff.
- Cup the fingers of your dominant hand, and carefully slide it into the glove.
- If the glove needs adjustments, wait until both gloves are on before making them.
- Using your dominant hand in the sterile glove, slide your fingers beneath the cuff of the remaining glove.
- Carefully slide the fingers of your nondominant hand into the glove.
- Make any necessary adjustments.
- Do not touch any non-sterile surfaces, and keep your hands above your waist to maintain sterility.

## Five Vital Signs

The five vital signs that are most commonly measured are temperature, pulse, respiration rate, blood pressure, and pain level.

1. Temperature measures the patient's core body temperature.
2. Pulse measures the number of times the patient's heart beats per minute.
3. Respiration rate measures the number of times the patient breathes every minute.
4. Blood pressure is recorded as two numbers. The top number is referred to as the systolic pressure; it measures the pressure within the patient's arteries during contraction of the heart. The bottom number is the diastolic blood pressure; this number reflects the pressure within the arteries while the heart is at rest between each contraction.
5. Pain level measures the presence or absence of pain. It indicates the severity of that pain according to the patient.

**Oral Temperature**

Wash your hands, don a pair of gloves, and greet the patient.

- Explain what you are going to do, and check the patient's armband.
- Ensure that the patient has not had anything to drink in the past 15 minutes as this will make his temperature read falsely low.
- Cover the thermometer with a plastic sheath, and place it under the patient's tongue.
- Instruct the patient to keep his mouth closed and not to talk while the thermometer is obtaining a reading.
- Wait until the thermometer indicates the temperature has been read.
- Note the temperature, clean the thermometer, remove your gloves, and wash your hands.

Axillary Temperature

Wash your hands, don a pair of gloves, and greet the patient.

- Explain what you are going to do, and verify the patient's identity by checking his armband.
- Make sure that the area under the patient's arm is dry.
- Place a plastic sheath over the temperature probe.
- Position the thermometer in the axillary area, and instruct the patient to keep his arm down.
- Leave the thermometer in place until it indicates a reading.
- If a mercury thermometer is being used, allow the thermometer to remain in place for 10 minutes.
- Record the temperature, remove the gloves, wash your hands, and clean the thermometer prior to using it on another patient.

Rectal Temperature

Wash your hands, don a pair of gloves, greet the patient, and explain what you are going to do. Identify the patient using his armband.

- Place a plastic cover over the temperature probe.
- Assist the patient into a side lying position.
- Apply lubrication to the thermometer, and slide it 1 inch into the patient's rectum.
- Leave it in place until a temperature reads.
- If you are using a mercury thermometer, leave it in place for 3 minutes.
- Remove the thermometer, and inspect it to make sure it is still intact.
- Record the temperature.
- Position the patient for comfort.
- Clean the thermometer, remove the gloves, and wash your hands.

*Indications of an abnormal temperature:*

A person's core body temperature is closely regulated to ensure an optimum environment for the complex chemical reactions within the body. The normal temperature range for an adult patient is between 97.8 and 99.1 degrees Fahrenheit.

A low core body temperature may indicate the onset of an infection. The patient's temperature may also be low after coming from a cold environment, such as the operating room.

The primary cause for an elevated temperature is infection. Because a fever is the result of the immune system mounting a defense against an infection, it may not be necessary to treat the fever unless the temperature goes above 101.5 degrees Fahrenheit.

## Apical Pulse

An apical pulse measures the number of times the heart beats every minute by auscultating at the apex of the heart.

- Wash your hands, greet the patient, and explain what you are going to do.
- Verify the patient's identity using his armband.
- Place the bell of the stethoscope against the patient's left chest and locate the area in which the pulse is the loudest.
- If the patient's heart rate is regular, count the number of beats for 30 seconds and multiply by two. If the patient's heart rate is irregular, count the number of beats for a full minute.
- Record the patient's pulse, clean the stethoscope, and wash your hands.

## Peripheral Pulse

Wash your hands, greet the patient, and explain what you are going to do.

- Check the patient's identity using his armband.
- Take the patient's hand, and slide your index and middle finger along the thumb, up to the hollow of the wrist.
- Apply gentle pressure until you can feel the pulse.
- If the patient's heart rate is regular, count the number of beats for 30 seconds and multiply that number by two.
- If the patient's heart rate is irregular, count the number of beats for a full minute. Record the number in the patient's chart.
- Wash your hands.

### Indications of an Abnormal Pulse

The normal pulse range for an adult is between 60 and 80 beats per minute. The patient may have a low heart rate if he is physically fit or if he is resting. Some medications may also decrease the patient's heart rate. An elevated heart rate may be the result of exercise, stress, drugs, or caffeine. Certain medications may also elevate the patient's heart rate. If the patient has an elevated temperature or an infection, the heart rate will be elevated. An elevated heart rate can also be the result of uncontrolled bleeding.

## Patient's Respirations

Measuring respirations is done to assess the number of times per minute the patient breathes. Typically, when a person is made aware of his breathing, he does not breathe deeply or regularly. Do not tell the patient you are measuring the respiration rate, as it will make him aware of his breathing and may produce an inaccurate result. The ideal time to measure the patient's respiration rate is after checking the patient's pulse. Count the number of times the patient breathes, counting one rise and fall of the chest wall as one respiration. Count the number of breaths for one minute, noting the depth of the breath and any use of accessory muscles. Record the respiratory rate on the patient's chart. Wash your hands.

<u>Indications of Abnormal Respirations</u>

The normal range for respiration rate is between 12 to 18 breaths per minute. A number of factors may affect the rate of the patient's breathing. The patient may breathe more slowly if he is resting or if he is positioned on his back. Certain narcotics may also depress the respiratory drive, resulting in fewer breaths per minute. A rapid respiration rate may be caused by increased activity, pain, or stress. An elevated temperature or an infection may cause the patient's respiratory rate to be quicker. Other conditions, such as respiratory distress, fluid overload, or a heart attack, may also cause an elevated respiratory rate.

## Patient's Blood Pressure

Wash your hands, greet the patient, and explain what you are going to do.

- Verify the patient's identity using his armband.
- Wrap the blood pressure cuff around the patient's upper arm, and place the bell of the stethoscope over the brachial artery.
- Pump the bulb of the blood pressure cuff, inflating the cuff between 150 and 180 mmHg.
- Slowly release the pressure, while listening through the stethoscope.
- Note the pressure at which you first hear a pulse; this is the systolic blood pressure.
- Continue to listen to the pulse.
- Note the pressure at which the pulse fades away; this is the patient's diastolic blood pressure.
- Record the findings on the patient's chart, and wash your hands.

<u>Orthostatic Blood Pressure</u>

Orthostatic hypotension is a condition in which the patient's blood pressure drops as a result of a change in position. This can cause dizziness or lightheadedness after standing, which may lead to falls. To check for orthostatic hypotension:

- Measure the patient's blood pressure while he is lying down.
- Assist the patient into a sitting position, and measure the blood pressure again.
- If the patient is able to stand, assist him into a standing position and measure the blood pressure a third time.
- If the patient's blood pressure drops by more than 20 mmHg systolic or 10 mmHg diastolic, then he is considered to have orthostatic hypotension. The nurse should be notified immediately.

<u>Abnormal Blood Pressure Indications</u>

The normal range for a systolic blood pressure is 110 to 140. The normal range for a diastolic blood pressure is 60 to 90. Hypotension is defined as a systolic blood pressure less than 100 mmHg. The patient may have a low blood pressure because he is resting or as a result of certain medications. Bleeding, infection, heart failure, or dehydration may also result in hypotension. Hypertension is defined as a systolic blood pressure greater than 150 mmHg. The patient may have hypertension as a result of chronic illness, pain, or stress. Hypertension may also be caused by kidney failure, heart disease, or certain neurological disorders.

## Intravenous Therapy

An intravenous (IV) line is a small tube that pierces the patient's skin and rests in the vein. It serves as a method of providing the patient with medication and fluids. While receiving IV therapy, the

- 57 -

patient should be closely monitored to make sure the IV line is in place. If the IV is leaking or oozing at the site, it may be an indication that the hub is not properly connected. If the patient complains of pain from the IV site coupled with warmth, redness, or swelling, it may be a sign that the IV line is no longer in the vein. All of these signs should be reported to the nurse.

## Measuring the Patient's Intake

In order to measure a patient's intake, the nurse aide must measure any liquids the patient takes in over a 24-hour period. This includes any water, milk, and juice the patient might drink, as well as any foods that melt at room temperature, such as ice cream, pudding, or jello. While measuring intake, the nurse aide should also include any tube feeding or any fluid that is used to flush a nasogastric tube. If the patient is receiving IV therapy, all IV fluids and medications suspended in IV fluid should be included in the patient's total intake. IV intake should also include any IV fluids that the patient received during surgery. Intake should be calculated in milliliters (mL) and added up over a 24-hour period. That total should then be reported to the nurse.

## Measuring Patient's Output

Output measures the amount of fluid the patient excretes during a 24-hour period. All urine should be measured prior to being discarded. The amount of liquid stool in a bedpan should be estimated prior to being discarded. If the patient has a nasogastric tube to wall suction, the nurse aide should note how much drainage the patient has had out of the tube. If the patient has a wound that is hooked to suction, note how much blood has been removed from the wound. If the patient is having drainage out of a wound that is not to suction, the nurse aide should note how many times the dressing needs to be changed. Estimated blood loss from surgery should also be included as output. Add all secretions over a 24-hour period, and make a note of it on the patient's chart.

## Observing the Patient's Bowel Movements

After the patient moves his bowel the nursing aide should make careful note of the color and character of the stool. If the patient has multiple bouts of diarrhea, the nurse should be notified as this places the patient at risk of developing dehydration. Dark, tarry stools indicate the patient may be bleeding within the intestinal tract. Frank blood should also be reported. Furthermore, if the patient has not had a bowel movement in more than three days, the nurse should be notified as this places the patient at risk for developing constipation.

*Intake and output calculation:* After intake and output have been calculated over a 24-hour period, the two numbers should be compared. Ideally, intake should equal output as this indicates an equal fluid balance. Too much intake puts the patient at a risk for fluid overload, while too much output puts the patient at risk for dehydration. After comparing intake and output over a 24-hour period, the nurse aide should compare intake and output over the past few days. This gives a better indication of the patient's ongoing fluid status. For example, a high intake on one day may be compensated on the following day with a high output, placing the patient's fluid balance at an equal level.

## Patient's Height and Weight

An upright scale can be used to measure the patient's height and weight if he has the strength to stand on the scale.

- Wash your hands, greet the patient, and explain what you are going to do.
- Confirm the patient's identity using his armband.
- Assist the patient to a standing position, and show him to the upright scale.

- Instruct the patient to stand on the scale, facing away from the scale.
- Lower the height rod until it rests on top of the patient's head.
- Make a note of the height.
- Assist the patient in turning until he is facing the scale.
- Move the weights on the scale until the bar is balanced; make a note of the patient's weight.
- Assist the patient back to the chair or bed, and position him for comfort.
- Wash your hands.

## Patient Lying in Bed

A patient who is bed bound will need to have his height and weight measured while in bed.

- Wash your hands, greet the patient, and explain what you are going to do.
- Verify the patient's identity using his armband.
- Obtain assistance from a colleague.
- Roll the patient onto a bath blanket and the bed scale pad.
- Prior to obtaining the weight, mark the placement of the patient's heels and the top of his head on the bath blanket.
- Weigh the patient using the bed scale, and make a note of the patient's weight.
- Remove the bed scale pad and the bath blanket.
- Measure the distance between the two marks on the pad, and record that as the patient's height.
- Reposition the patient for comfort, and wash your hands.

## Observations of Patient

While interacting with a patient, the nurse aide must be vigilant to observe any changes in the patient's mental status. Check to see if the patient is alert or if he appears to be difficult to awaken. Assess the patient for any signs of confusion, such as disorientation to place or time. Make a note of any changes, such as increased weakness, slurring of speech, or the inability to follow commands. If the patient shows any of these signs, the nurse should be notified immediately as these may indicate severe physical or neurological problems.

## Data Collection and Reporting

If a change in the patient's status has occurred, the nurse aide should notify the patient's nurse immediately. The information should be reported in a succinct manner. The patient's name, as well as the room number and the bed number, should be included in the report. The nature of the problem should be explained, including the time of onset. The nurse aide should report any observations that accompany the problem. For example, if the patient developed confusion two hours ago, the nurse aide should include the manner in which the patient is confused.

## Objective and Subjective Data

Objective data refers to information that can be referred to as fact. Objective data is quantifiable, such as vital signs, the patient's weight, or intake and output. Objective data also refers to anything that can be observed by another person. For example, if the patient has flushed cheeks, this is considered to be an objective fact.

Subjective data refers to anything the patient thinks or feels. The patient's pain level is subjective.

For example, the patient is developing a urinary tract infection. Objective data concerning that fact may be observations concerning cloudiness of the patient's urine. Meanwhile, patient's complaints of pain and difficulty urinating would be considered subjective data.

## Charting Purposes

The purpose of charting is to create an accurate log regarding the care given to the patient, as well as the patient's response to the care. Items typically included in the chart are vital signs, intake and output, assessments, and procedure notes. Assessments are typically recorded on preprinted forms; any abnormalities in the patient's assessment are included in the narrative notes. This is referred to as charting by exception. Notes are made in the patient's chart any time a procedure is performed on the patient. Most information included should be objective in nature. Whether or not the nurse aide makes narrative notes in the chart is dependent upon hospital policy.

### Charting Principals

While writing in the patient's chart write with only blue or black ink. Do not use a pencil. Write legibly, including only objective information. Avoid speculating or becoming overly emotional in the note. If an error is made, draw a single line through the erroneous information. Over the erroneous information, write "Error", the reason for the error, and your initials. Do not scratch out or scribble over the mistake. Do not use correction fluid to cover any errors. Do not edit another person's note or write over another person's writing.

# Basic Nursing Skills

## Shaving a Patient

Prior to beginning the procedure; wash your hands, greet the patient, and explain what you are going to do.

- Apply a pair of gloves, and use a wet washcloth to moisten the hair on the patient's face and neck.
- Check the razor to make sure it does not have any loose blades or jagged edges.
- Drape the patient with a towel, and apply shaving cream to the area that needs to be shaved.
- Use one hand to pull the skin taut, while moving the razor with firm strokes in the direction that the hair is growing.
- Rinse the razor in a basin of water as often as necessary.
- Use a moistened washcloth to rinse off all remaining shaving cream.

## Performing Hair Care on a Patient

Prior to beginning hair care on the patient, wash your hands, greet the patient, and explain what you are going to do.

- Don a pair of gloves.
- Raise the head of the bed to a comfortable level, and place a towel beneath the patient's head.
- Part the patient's hair into manageable sections, and run the comb or brush slowly through it.
- If the hair is tangled, hold the strand of hair above the tangle while combing it to prevent pulling the patient's hair. As you are combing, carefully inspect the scalp for any lesions, lice, or signs of dryness.
- Try to shape the hair into the patient's preferred style; even parting the hair on the correct side can provide a greater level of comfort for the patient. After hair care is complete, remove the towel and reposition the patient for comfort.

## Nail Care

Prior to beginning nail care, wash your hands, greet the patient, and explain what you are going to do.

- Don a pair of gloves.
- Soak the patient's hands in warm water to soften them and prevent the nails from cracking.
- Carefully remove any dirt from beneath the patient's nails.
- Trim each nail by cutting straight across with a pair of nail clippers, then round the edges using an emery board.
- Be careful not to cut the nails too short as this may cause irritation to the nail bed.
- If desired, apply lotion to the patient's nails.
- After nail care has been completed, reposition the patient for comfort and wash your hands.

## Oral Care

Oral care performed on an unconscious patient as follows:

- Prior to beginning oral care on an unconscious patient, wash your hands, check the patient's name band, and explain what you are going to do.
- Don a pair of gloves, and drape a towel over the patient's chest.
- Adjust the level of the bed to a comfortable height, and raise the head of the bed greater than 30 degrees.
- Turn the patient's head toward you, and hold the mouth open with a tongue depressor in one hand.
- Clean the patient's teeth, gums, and tongue.
- After cleaning has been completed, suction the secretions out of the patient's mouth.
- Position the patient for comfort, remove the gloves, and wash your hands.

Oral care performed on a conscious patient as follows:

- Some patients may be unable to perform oral care on themselves as a result of palsy or weakness in the upper extremities.
- Before beginning oral care, wash your hands, greet the patient, and explain what you are going to do.
- Don a pair of gloves, and drape a towel over the patient.
- Raise the level of the bed to a comfortable height, and position the head of the bed greater than 30 degrees.
- Using a toothbrush, thoroughly clean the patient's teeth, gums, and tongue.
- While performing oral care, carefully inspect the patient's mouth for any lesions or signs of infection.
- If the patient is able to take small amounts of water without aspirating, allow him to rinse his mouth and spit the water into an emesis basin.
- Position the patient for comfort, and wash your hands.

Denture care is performed as follows:

- Prior to beginning denture care, wash your hands, greet the patient, and explain what you are going to do.
- Don a pair of gloves, and obtain the patient's dentures.
- Place a towel or washcloth in the sink to prevent breakage if the dentures are accidentally dropped.
- Using a toothbrush, clean the surface of the patient's dentures.
- Place them in a denture cup filled with cool water.
- Provide oral care to the patient using sponge swabs and mouthwash; carefully observe for any lesions or signs of infection.
- After the procedure has been completed, position the patient for comfort and wash your hands.

## Bathing

Process for performing a bed bath as follows:

- Prior to beginning the bed bath, wash your hands, greet the patient, and explain what you are going to do.
- Fill a basin with water at a temperature between 105 and 115 degrees, and remove as much medical equipment as possible.
- Keep the patient covered to maintain dignity.
- Allow the patient to bathe as much of himself as possible.
- Begin by washing the patient's face, moving downward to the arms, the chest, abdomen, legs, back, and perineal area.
- Use a different washcloth for each area of the body.
- If necessary, change the patient's bed linens while washing the back.
- Apply lotion if desired.
- After the bath has been completed, reposition the patient for comfort and wash your hands.

Procedures for performing a tub bath as follows:

- Prior to beginning the tub bath, wash your hands, greet the patient, and explain what you are going to do.
- Make sure the bathtub has been cleaned.
- Place towels in the tub and on the floor outside the tub to prevent slipping.
- Ambulate the patient to the tub, observing all precautions.
- Once the patient is in the tub, fill it to the desired level.
- Make sure the water temperature is about 115 degrees.
- Provide privacy while the patient washes, but maintain close supervision to make sure the patient does not slip.
- Wash the patient's back and any area he is unable to reach.
- Drain the water, and dry the patient.
- Assist the patient into a standing position, and carefully help him out of the tub.
- Assist the patient in putting on his clothes.
- Position the patient for comfort, clean the tub, and wash your hands.

Procedure for perineal care as follows:

- Perineal care is an important part of bathing because it allows the nurse aide to inspect the skin of the perineal area. If done properly, it also decreases the risk for urinary tract infections.
- Perineal care should be done during a complete bath and should also be performed after the patient is incontinent.
- Wash your hands, and don a pair of gloves.
- Instruct the patient to open his legs.
- Cleanse the skin of the perineal area, using front to back movements.
- Never wash from back to front as this can introduce germs from the anus to the urethral area. After the skin has been cleansed, completely dry the area.
- Do not reuse the linens used to wash the peri area.
- Obtain a clean towel and washcloth to finish the bath.

**Back Rub Procedure**

Prior to giving a backrub:

- Wash your hands, greet the patient, and explain what you are going to do.
- Ensure that privacy is provided, and don a pair of gloves.
- If necessary, wash the patient's back with warm water and dry it completely.
- Warm the lotion in the basin of water, and apply a small amount to your hands. \
- Begin the backrub at the small of the patient's back, and work your way toward the shoulders using long, firm strokes.
- Use a circular motion when rubbing over bony areas to prevent irritating the skin.
- While performing the backrub, carefully observe the patient's skin for any signs of breakdown.
- After the back rub has been completed, position the patient for comfort and wash your hands.

**Making an Unoccupied Bed**

The linens on an unoccupied bed can be changed whenever the patient is out of bed.

- Wash your hands, and raise the level of the bed to a comfortable height.
- Lower all of the side rails.
- Place the fitted sheet on the bed, and pull it tight to make sure it does not wrinkle.
- Place the pad on the bed so that it will be positioned below the patient's hips and lower back.
- Carefully unfold the flat sheet, and place it on the bed, tucking the blanket so that the edges are mitered.
- Place the blanket on the bed, and fold the lower edge so that the corners are mitered.
- Fold the blanket and sheet back over the foot of the bed.
- Raise the side rails on one side of the bed, and put the bed back into the lowest position.
- Wash your hands.

Mitered Corners

Mitered corners on a hospital bed prevent the sheet from being easily removed from the bottom of the bed.

- Place the sheet on the bed, and make sure there is an equal length of fabric hanging over each edge.
- Tuck the short end of the bottom edge below the mattress.
- Grasp one of the lower corners of the sheet and pull it taut.
- Pull it upward and at an angle toward the head of the bed so that it creates a triangle on top of the sheet.
- While keeping the corner taunt, grasp the edge that is hanging over the side and tuck it beneath the mattress.
- Release the corner and allow it to fall into place, and then tuck the remaining fabric beneath the mattress.

<u>Making an Occupied Bed</u>

While the patient is turned on his side, undo the dirty fitted sheet and roll it toward the patient, placing the side that touched the patient inside the rolled up linen.

- Unfold the clean fitted sheet, and place it on the half of the bed that has been unmade.
- Place the pad on the bed so that it will be positioned beneath the patient's hips.
- Roll the clean linen, and tuck it beneath the rolled dirty linen.
- Turn the patient over the rolled up linen, onto the other side.
- Remove the dirty fitted sheet and pad, and place them in the soiled linen container.
- Unroll the clean fitted sheet and pad, pulling taut to ensure there are no wrinkles.
- Secure the fitted sheet to the bed. Roll the patient onto his back.
- Cover the patient with a sheet and blanket, and then miter the lower corners.
- Position the patient for comfort.

## Indwelling Catheter

An indwelling or Foley catheter is typically placed in patients who are unable to completely empty their bladder while voiding. It may also be placed for incontinent patients to protect their skin from the acidity of the urine. Post-surgical or critical care patients may receive an indwelling catheter in order to accurately measure their urinary output. The indwelling catheter is placed using sterile technique as follows:

- A rubber tube is threaded up the patient's urethra and into the bladder.
- A bulb at the end of the tube is inflated using sterile water; this keeps the tube in place and prevents leakage around the catheter.
- An indwelling catheter places the patient at an increased risk of developing a urinary tract infection.
- Catheter care should be performed frequently, and the catheter should be removed as soon as possible.

<u>Caring for a Patient</u>

Greet the patient, and explain what you are going to do.

- Wash your hands, and don a pair of gloves.
- Place the patient in a supine position, and lower the head of the bed.
- Place a water-resistant pad beneath the patient's hips.
- Using warm water, wash around the urethra in a downward circular motion.
- Never wash in an upward motion, as this may introduce germs from the rectum to the catheter.
- Wash around the indwelling catheter tube to remove any sediment that might be present.
- Carefully dry the patient's peri area.
- Hang the bag so that it is below the bladder, and make sure there are no kinks in the tubing.
- Never let the catheter bag touch the floor, as this can introduce germs into the bag and catheter tubing.
- Make sure the tubing is secured to the patient's inner thigh to prevent the tube from tugging.
- Once the procedure is done, remove the pad and cover the patient.
- Remove your gloves, and wash your hands.

*Patient with an indwelling catheter:*

When a patient has an indwelling catheter, the urine should be checked frequently.

- The amount of urine drained from the catheter should be noted and reported to the patient's nurse.
- If the patient is not urinating enough (less than 30mLs per hour) or too much (greater than 400mLs per hour), the nurse should be notified.
- The appearance of the urine should also be monitored, and any abnormalities should be reported.
- Abnormal findings include cloudiness, sediment in the urine, or an unusual color, such as dark amber or green.
- The nurse should also be notified if the patient's urine is blood-tinged or foul smelling.

## Placing a Patient on the Bedpan

Wash your hands, and greet the patient.

- Explain what you are going to do.
- Make sure the patient has privacy, and put on a pair of gloves.
- Lay the patient flat in a supine position, and turn him on his side.
- Place the bedpan over the buttocks, and carefully roll him back onto his back.
- Instruct the patient to open his legs, and make sure the bedpan has been placed properly.
- Raise the head of the bed, give the patient the call bell, and instruct the patient to call when finished.
- Remove your gloves, and wash your hands.

Getting the Patient off of the Bedpan

When the patient is ready to get off the bedpan:

- Ensure the patient has privacy.
- Wash your hands, and don a pair of gloves.
- Lay the head of the bed flat, and turn the patient on his side.
- While turning the patient, support the bedpan in order to prevent secretions from leaking into the bed.
- Remove the bedpan, and set it to one side.
- Provide perineal care for the patient.
- Position the patient for comfort, and allow him to wash his hands with a damp rag, if desired.
- Measure the output, and dispose of the secretions.

## Providing Patient with a Meal Tray

Before taking the tray into the patient's room:

- Nursing aide should check to make sure the patient is receiving the correct tray.
- Check the patient's armband and compare it to the name and room number on the tray.
- Check to make sure the patient's tray contains foods that are appropriate for the patient's ordered diet.

- Raise the patient's head of the bed, and place a towel over him to prevent bits of food from falling into bed.
- If the patient requires further assistance, cut any large pieces of food into bite-size pieces and open any containers.

## Feeding a Patient

Wash your hands, and raise the head of the patient's bed.

- Explain to the patient what foods are being served on the tray, and allow the patient to select what foods he will be fed first.
- When providing a bite to the patient, ensure the spoon is only half full.
- Use only the tip of the spoon to feed him.
- Feed the patient slowly, ensuring the patient has swallowed all of the food in his mouth before offering the next bite.
- Make sure the patient has had enough food to eat before taking the tray away.
- If the patient appears to be having difficulty swallowing, stop feeding the patient immediately and notify the nurse.

*Tasks to be performed after assisting the patient with eating are as follows:* After the patient has finished eating, remove the meal tray and calculate the amount of food the patient took in.

- If the patient is on a calorie count diet, calculate the percentage of food eaten and tolerance to the food.
- If the patient's intake and output is being monitored, calculate the amount of fluid the patient took in.
- Report these findings to the nurse.
- Position the patient for comfort, and place the call light within reach.
- Make sure any necessary items, such as the tray table and personal items are within reach.
- Hand hygiene should then be performed.

*Indications that the patient is not swallowing properly are as follows:*
- A helpless patient is at a significant risk for aspirating food.
- During aspiration, small amounts of food and water move down the trachea and into the patient's lungs.
- Forceful coughing or a wet-sounding voice after swallowing a bite of food may be an indication of aspiration.
- If a patient needs to chew food for long periods of time or requires multiple attempts to swallow food, he may be aspirating.
- Other indications include unusual head movements while trying to swallow, difficulty breathing, drooling while eating, or pocketing food in the cheeks.

All of these signs should be reported to the patient's nurse.

## Applying Elastic Bandages

Prior to applying an elastic bandage, check the order to confirm where the bandage is to be placed.

- Wash your hands, greet the patient, and explain what you are going to do. Apply a pair of gloves.
- Hold the end of the bandage in place with one hand, and wrap it around the extremity twice to secure it.
- Continue to wrap the bandage around the area that needs to be covered, working from bottom to top.
- While wrapping, overlap the bandages to keep them from sliding down and to ensure the area is covered.
- Once the elastic bandage is in place, secure it with tape, clips, or Velcro.
- Remove the gloves, and wash your hands.

## Applying Anti-Embolism Stockings

Prior to applying anti-embolism stockings:

- Wash your hands, greet the patient, and explain what you are going to do.
- Verify the anti-embolism stockings are the proper size for the patient based upon height and weight; they should be tight without cutting off circulation.
- Place the patient in a supine position.
- Gather the fabric of the anti-embolism stocking and slide it onto the patient's foot.
- Roll the stocking upward until the upper edge is placed above the patient's knee.
- Check to make sure there are no wrinkles in the stocking and that the stocking is placed properly so that the toes and heels are in the appropriate spots.
- Once the stocking is in place, position the patient for comfort, remove your gloves, and wash your hands.

*Patients who are wearing elastic bandages or anti-embolism stockings:* While patients are wearing anti-embolism stockings or elastic bandages, it is important to monitor them closely to ensure they receive an appropriate amount of circulation to their extremities.

- Frequently assess the patient's toes (or fingers, if the elastic bandage is on the arm) to check for signs of decreased circulation.
- Any complaints of numbness, tingling, or decreased sensation in the extremity should be reported to the nurse and investigated immediately.
- Make sure to remove the patient's anti-embolism stockings every 8 hours to allow for circulation.
- Elastic bandages should be removed per the doctor's order.

## Range of Motion on Patients

Patients who are bed bound are at an increased risk of muscle deterioration from lack of use. Lack of regular exercise also places patients at risk for developing contractures, a painful condition that results in the permanent shortening of the muscle or tendon. Range-of-motion exercises can be performed to maintain muscle tone during periods in which the patient lacks the strength to perform other forms of activity. Patients may also be assisted with performing range-of-motion activities if they are unable to do so themselves, such as in cases in which patients are sedated or comatose.

## AROM and PROM

Active range of motion (AROM) occurs when patients are able to perform range-of-motion activities by themselves. Though they may receive directions from the nurse aide, patients perform the bulk of the exercise.

Passive range of motion (PROM) consists of the same exercises that are performed during AROM. PROM occurs when the nurse aide is performing range-of-motion activities on a sedated or comatose patient to prevent muscle weakness. PROM may also be performed on patients whose muscle weakness is so pronounced that they require assistance in order to perform the activity.

## Flexion

Flexion refers to bending at a joint, resulting in a decrease in the angle of the joint.

## Extension

Extension refers to the straightening of a joint, or increasing the angle of that joint. For example, when the arm is bent at the elbow, it is flexed. When the arm is straightened, it is extended.

## Adduction

Adduction refers to the movement away from the trunk. Adduction refers to a movement that brings a limb closer to the trunk. When the arm is moved away from the body, such as during jumping jacks, it is abducted. When it moves back toward the body, it is adducted.

## Rotation

Rotation occurs when a part of the body pivots on a central axis. When the head turns from side to side, it is considered to be rotating.

## Performing Range of Motion on a Patient

Range-of-motion exercises are typically performed during the patient's bath. They can be performed while the patient is sitting in a chair or lying in bed. Each exercise should be performed 10 times to ensure it is effective.

- Wash your hands, and explain to the patient what you are going to do.
- Raise the level of the bed until it is a comfortable height for you.
- Begin by performing range-of-motion exercises on the patient's head; instruct the patient to rotate his head from one side to the other.
- This exercise should not be performed on patients who have suffered neck or spinal cord injuries.
- Work on the arms next.
- Flex and extend both arms at the elbow, then abduct and adduct the arm.
- Flex and extend both wrists and all fingers.
- Range of motion of the legs includes flexion and extension of the leg at the knee, as well as abduction and adduction of the leg.
- Finally, flex and extend the ankles and toes.

*Abnormal findings to be reported if discovered while performing range-of-motion exercises:* Range-of-motion exercises should be performed at least once or twice every day to make sure the patient's joints do not become contracted.

- Stiffness or the inability to move the joint may be an indication of the onset of contractures; if either of these symptoms is noticed, they should be reported to the nurse immediately.

- While performing range of motion, the nursing aide should monitor for any signs of swelling or inflammation in the joints.
- If the patient experiences sudden severe pain or respiratory distress while performing range of motion, the nurse should be notified immediately.
  - Supine position: when the patient is in a supine position, he is lying flat on the back, with arms extended at the sides.
  - Prone position: a prone position consists of the patient resting on the stomach, with the head turned to one side on the pillow and arms extended at the side.
  - Lateral position; when the patient is in the lateral position, he should be positioned on his side, with both legs straight.
  - Sims' position: Sims' position is similar to the lateral position in that the patient is lying on the side. However, in the Sims' position, the patient's topmost leg is flexed. Both the flexed leg and topmost arm are elevated on a pillow for additional support.
  - Semi –Fowler Position: the semi-Fowler's position consists of the patient lying on the back with the head of the bed at a 45-degree angle.
  - High Fowler: a high-Fowler's position is similar to the semi-Fowler, however, the head of the bed is raised to a 90-degree angle.

## Placing the Patient in a Side-Lying Position

Wash your hands, don a pair of gloves, and explain to the patient what you are going to do.

- Obtain assistance to help turn the patient.
- Raise the level of the bed to a comfortable height.
- Using the draw sheet, move the patient closer to the side of the bed opposite of the direction you intend to turn him; this will allow the patient to remain in the center of the bed after having been turned.
- Grasp the draw sheet and use it to pull the patient onto his side.
- If the patient is able, ask him to grasp the side rail while you position him.
- Tuck a pillow beneath the patient's back, under the draw sheet.
- Tuck another pillow beneath the patient's buttocks.
- Place a pillow underneath the patient's arm and between the patient's knees for support.
- Remove your gloves, and wash your hands.

## Logrolling Procedure

Logrolling is a procedure that is performed whenever the patient has sustained a neck or spinal cord injury. Ideally, patients with this type of injury should be turned as little as possible until the neck or spine has been stabilized. In certain cases, turning cannot be avoided, such as if the patient has become incontinent. If the patient must be moved, the head, neck, and back must be kept in a stable position to prevent further injury. This requires good communication among the caregivers who are moving the patient to ensure that their movements are coordinated to maintain proper alignment. Logrolling a patient requires a minimum of three people in order to be performed successfully.

- Wash your hands, don a pair of gloves, and explain what you are going to do.
- Have one person positioned at the patient's head, and two others on the side in which the patient is to be facing.
- Grasp the draw sheet, and turn the patient.
- The person at the head of the bed should keep the patient's head midline with the rest of the body, while the people at the side of the bed keep the back and hips in alignment.

- Perform the necessary procedures, and then return the patient to his back.
- It is imperative that the patient's head, neck, and back are kept in alignment.
- Position the patient for comfort, and wash your hands.

# Role and Responsibility

## Patient's Responsibilities

The health care facility must make every reasonable effort to provide treatment for the patient. However, an optimal level of health cannot be achieved without the assistance of the patient. The patient must actively participate in his care in order for treatment to be successful. Much like the patient's Bill of Rights, the list of Patient Responsibilities should be provided to the patient on admission to the health care facility. These responsibilities include honesty and respect for health care providers, compliance with the treatment plan, meeting financial obligations, not putting others at risk, and responsible decision making. Failure to perform these responsibilities may result in the inability of the health care facility to provide adequate treatment. It is the patient's right to expect his health care providers to behave in a manner that is polite and respectful; the patient also has a responsibility to behave in a manner that is respectful toward his health care providers.

Hospitalization is a stressful time for a patient; however, it does not excuse disrespectful behavior. Swearing, sexual harassment, and violence are unacceptable behaviors. Acting in such a way makes it difficult for the health care team to provide adequate care. If the patient exhibits behavior that is inappropriate, it should be addressed immediately to make sure it does not interfere with his care. It is also important for the patient to be honest when interacting with the health care staff. The patient should be forthright when answering questions regarding medical and social history as this information is vital in planning the patient's care. Without all of the necessary information, the planned treatment may be inadequate or may cause harm to the patient.

## Health Habits

The key to maintaining a quality lifestyle is maintaining healthy habits. Healthy habits include a proper diet, exercise, and appropriate lifestyle choices. Though members of the health care team can provide information and encouragement regarding a healthy lifestyle, only the patient can make the necessary changes.

It is the responsibility of the health care staff to review the treatment plan and provide education regarding necessary lifestyle changes. However, the treatment is only effective as long as the patient is compliant.

If the patient chooses to refuse to follow the treatment plan, he must take responsibility if the plan were to fail. It is the patient's right to determine the type of care he receives. While it is the responsibility of the health care team to provide adequate information to allow the patient to make a decision regarding treatment, it is the patient's responsibility to make that decision responsibly. If there is an aspect of the treatment plan that is unclear, the patient should ask questions in order to seek clarification. It is also the patient's responsibility to make decisions regarding treatment based upon the information that has been provided to him, rather than basing his decision on emotions.

## Standards of Care

Standards of care provide a guideline that explains how a nursing aide is expected to act in a given situation. The state government or the health care facility in which the nursing aide is practicing typically sets these standards.

- It is the responsibility of the nursing aide to be aware of the appropriate standards of care.
- If the nursing aide were to fail to act appropriately in a given situation, she could be held responsible for any harm that might come to the patient as a result of her deviating from the expected way to practice.

## Scope of Practice

Scope of practice is a list of tasks that a nursing aide is allowed to perform as determined by the state certification board. It is the responsibility of the nursing aide to be aware of what tasks she can and cannot perform. Any activity that does not appear on the list falls outside the nursing aide's scope of practice; if the nursing aide is caught performing an activity that is not on the list, she runs the risk of losing her certification. The nursing aide is liable for any harm that comes to the patient as a result of the nursing aide performing an activity that is outside her scope of practice.

### Tasks Not Part of the Nursing Aide's Scope of Practice

There are a number of tasks that fall outside the nursing aide's scope of practice. A nursing aide is not allowed to receive orders from a doctor; only a nurse can write orders. A nursing aide may not insert or remove devices from a patient's body, such as indwelling catheters, IVs, or rectal tubes. Also, a nursing aide may not perform any sort of sterile procedure. In most cases, a nursing aide may not administer medications. Some states allow a nursing aide to assist the patient in self-administration of medication under specific circumstances. The nursing aide may only assist in medication administration if she receives special training and may only assist in administering certain medications.

### Nursing Aide Procedures When Asked to Perform out of Her Scope of Practice

If a nursing aide feels she is being asked to perform an assignment that is outside of her scope of practice, she should talk to the charge nurse privately after the assignments have been given. The nursing aide should explain why she feels uncomfortable about the assignment. If necessary, the facility's policy and procedure manual can be consulted to confirm if the assigned task falls within the nursing aide's scope of practice. If it does, and the nursing aide still feels uncomfortable, she should request that the charge nurse be present while the task is being performed to ensure it is performed correctly.

## Liability

Liability refers to the responsibility of a person to act within the confines of the law. In the eyes of the law, a person must take responsibility for his own actions.

If a nursing aide fails to perform a task to the best of her ability and harm comes to the patient, she can be considered liable. Similarly, if the nursing aide performs a task that falls outside of her scope of practice and harm comes to the patient, she is considered liable. In order to maintain safe practice, it is important for a nursing aide to perform tasks exactly as she learned them, without taking shortcuts. She should also make an effort to keep her skills and knowledge up to date with current health care trends.

## Behaving in an Ethical Manner

Behaving in an ethical manner refers to doing what is right. In order to provide ethically appropriate care, the nursing aide should strive to consistently provide high-quality care for her patients.

In order for a nursing aide to behave in an ethical manner, she must act in a manner that is in accordance with the standards of practice within her state. Behaving in an ethical manner also includes respecting the patient's rights, such as the right to privacy and confidentiality. Ethical behavior also includes remembering that not everyone behaves with the same values and ideals and respecting them for their differences.

> **Review Video: Organizational Ethics**
> Visit mometrix.com/academy and enter code: 885880
>
> **Review Video: Confidentiality**
> Visit mometrix.com/academy and enter code: 250384

## Civil and Criminal Law

There are two different types of court cases: civil cases and criminal cases.

1. Civil court cases take place between two people, when a wronged individual sues the person who did him wrong. If the accused is found guilty in a civil case, he is typically made to pay fines and restoration to the wronged party.
2. In a criminal court case, the defendant is accused of committing crimes against society as a whole. If a person is found guilty in a criminal case, he is made to pay fines or serve time in jail.

## A Tort

A tort is a wrong that is committed in a civil case. There are two types of torts: unintentional and intentional.

1. In an unintentional tort, a person commits a wrong against another person without intending to cause harm. For example, if a nursing aide forgets to put the side rails back up on the bed and the patient falls and injures himself as a result, that could be considered an unintentional tort.
2. An intentional tort occurs when a person has the intention of causing harm to another person. An example of an intentional tort is if the nursing aide leaves the unit without telling anybody, and the patient becomes injured while he is not being monitored.

## Assault

Assault refers to the threat or attempt to touch or inflict physical harm on another person. The threat could be verbal or physical, such as a threatening gesture or advancing toward a person in a threatening way. Caution must be taken while caring for a patient; if the patient refuses a treatment and the nursing aide attempts to force the patient to receive the treatment, she may be liable for assault. It is important to remember that the patient does not have to be harmed in order for the nursing aide to be found liable for assault. It is only necessary to prove that the patient felt threatened in a particular situation.

## Battery

Battery refers to the act of touching a person without permission. It could refer to a violent act or an unintended act. A nursing aide might also be accused of battery for performing a procedure on a patient without his consent. In order to protect herself from being accused of battery, a nursing aide should take a moment to explain the procedure to the patient prior to beginning and obtain consent from the patient to perform the procedure. If the patient refuses the procedure, the nursing aide should try to explain the reasons why the procedure is necessary but should not attempt to force the patient to have the procedure performed.

## Negligence

Negligence is the failure to perform care in the manner in which that person was trained. A nursing aide can be charged with negligence if she does not act in a way that is reasonable for a person with her level of training. For example, if the nursing aide leaves a patient unattended in the shower and the patient falls and injures himself, the nursing aide could be found negligent. A nursing aide can avoid being accused of negligence by performing procedures exactly as she learned how to do them, without taking shortcuts. If the nursing aide is unsure how to perform a procedure, she should not hesitate to ask for assistance.

### Reporting Negligent Behavior of a Co-Worker

The nursing aide should be observant for any signs of negligence in the health care facility. Negligence can include failing to perform important tasks, such as turning or ambulating, or performing patient care activities in a manner that is unsafe.

If the nursing aide sees another member of the health care team behaving in a way that is negligent, she should report that behavior to the charge nurse. If it is the charge nurse who is behaving negligently, the nursing aide should utilize the proper chain of command to make sure the behavior is addressed. She should not try to confront the negligent coworker herself.

## Defamation

When a person makes statements about another person that causes damage to the individual's reputation, she can be accused of defamation.

- Slander refers to spoken defamation. For example, if a nursing aide spreads rumors that a patient has HIV, that nursing aide can be accused of slander.
- Libel refers to a written statement that causes injury to another person's reputation. For example, if the nursing aide writes an article that a doctor is practicing without appropriate licensure and that article is untrue, she can be accused of libel.

A nursing aide can avoid being accused of slander by avoiding saying negative things about other people. By spreading rumors, the nursing aide is acting unprofessionally and places herself at risk for being accused of defamation.

## Malpractice

Malpractice is a type of negligence that is committed by a professional who needs to maintain a license in order to practice. In a case of malpractice, a professional fails to act according to standards of care within her profession, which results in harm coming to the patient. Malpractice is more severe than negligence; it takes into account the professional's higher level of training when considering the wrong that was committed by the health care professional. Nursing aides cannot be sued for malpractice as they are only required to maintain certification. However, they can still be sued for negligence.

## Invasion of Privacy

The patient has a right to keep details about him private. Invasion of privacy refers to failure to maintain the patient's right to privacy by relaying personal information without the patient's consent. The patient's privacy can be invaded if the nursing aide shares details about the patient's health history with others or by inadvertently leaving sensitive documents where others can easily see them.

A nursing aide can avoid being accused of invasion of privacy by only discussing details of the case with those who are directly involved in the care of the patient. If a person who is not part of the patient's immediate family wants information regarding the patient's treatment, the nursing aide should refer him to the charge nurse.

## Abandonment

Abandonment occurs when a nursing aide leaves without notifying others or securing another person to provide care in her place. If harm befalls a patient while the nursing aide is absent of her duties, she can be accused of abandonment. A nursing aide can avoid being accused of abandonment by asking another nursing aide to cover her patients and informing the charge nurse prior to leaving the unit. She should also make an effort to make sure all of her patients are safe and secure prior to giving report and leaving the unit.

## Fraud

When a person commits fraud, she deliberately misrepresents herself for personal gain. It can be considered a violation of either civil or criminal law.

A nursing aide would commit fraud if she claimed to be a nurse or a doctor in the presence of a patient. It is also considered fraud to lie about one's qualifications or certifications on a resume in order to secure a job. A nursing aide can avoid being accused of fraud by clearly identifying herself when dealing with a patient. She can also avoid being accused of fraud by acting within her scope of practice.

## Theft

Theft is the removal of another person's money or belongings without his knowledge. A nursing aide is guilty of theft if she takes a patient's belongings, even if the stolen item is not being used or is not of significant monetary value.

Though the health care facility takes steps to avoid hiring people who might steal from patients, the nursing aide should be vigilant as well. The nursing aide should try to avoid theft by not leaving the patient's belongings in plain sight when they are not in use. If she sees someone stealing a patient's belongings or acting suspiciously, she should report the behavior to the charge nurse immediately.

## False Imprisonment

False imprisonment refers to confining a person to an area against his will. It is typically used in reference to use of restraints. Restraints are an acceptable tool to be used as a last resort in order to protect both the patient and the safety of others.

False imprisonment refers to the use of restraints without an order or in a situation in which it is inappropriate to restrain the patient. A patient could also be falsely imprisoned if he is confined to the health care facility when he wishes to leave. If the patient expresses a desire to leave the hospital and he is alert and able to make decisions for himself, the nursing aide should avoid attempting to force the patient to stay. Instead, she should notify the charge nurse or the supervisor immediately.

## Abuse

Abuse is any sort of action that results in the physical harm, mental harm, or death of the patient. It is a criminal act and most typically results in imprisonment. Abusive actions can be deliberate or can be the result of negligence. It can take a number of forms, including physical, psychological, verbal, sexual, or financial abuse. Abuse can be subtle, and some victims of abuse may be reluctant to come forward. The nursing aide should be vigilant for any signs of abuse and report any findings to the charge nurse immediately.

### Psychological Abuse

Psychological or emotional abuse occurs when a person uses psychological attacks in order to intimidate or humiliate another person. It is typically done in order to coerce the person into doing something that he does not want to do. Psychological abuse can include teasing, threatening harm, or abandonment.

Psychological abuse can be difficult to identify because it does not necessarily leave physical marks. Person who has been psychologically abused may show vague symptoms, such as chronic depression, anxiety, anger, or posttraumatic stress disorder. In many cases, other types of abuse accompany psychological abuse.

### Verbal Abuse

Verbal abuse refers to using words and threats in order to demean or upset another person. Verbal abuse includes threatening another person, raising one's voice in anger, or using profanity or derogatory statements toward the other person.

It can be difficult to identify a person who is being verbally abused. They may complain of vague symptoms, such as depression, anxiety, anger, or a feeling of hopelessness. In many cases, the victim may blame himself or herself for the abuse or may be overcome with hopelessness that the abuse cannot be stopped. Verbal abuse is often accompanied by physical abuse.

### Financial Abuse

Financial abuse occurs when a person takes the money and belongings of another person. The elderly are most commonly the victims of financial abuse. Forms of financial abuse include forcing a person to sign over property, using monthly disability checks for items other than the elderly person's care, or forging another person's signature.

Being observant is the best way to catch financial abuse. It is possible that the patient is being abused financially if the patient lacks basic amenities, such as appropriate clothing or necessary personal items, (e.g. glasses or hearing aids) despite adequate financial assistance.

### Physical Abuse

Physical abuse is the most obvious form of abuse. It occurs when one person deliberately inflicts harm on another person and may be accompanied by verbal, emotional, or sexual abuse.

Signs of physical abuse include bruising or abrasions with a distinctive shape, such as a fist or foot. Any injuries that do not coincide with the provided explanation should be suspected. For example, a caregiver states that the patient burned himself while cooking. The explanation would be suspect if the burns are in a suspicious place, such as on the inner arm or on the abdomen. If a caregiver refuses to leave the patient's side during an interview or insists upon speaking for the patient, this behavior should also be suspected.

Sexual Abuse

Sexual abuse is any unwanted sexual behavior directed from one person to another. It includes any sexually suggestive comments or gestures, unwanted touching or fondling, or coercion to perform a sexual act. Additional forms of sexual abuse include sexual harassment or behavior that is sexually demeaning. Other forms of abuse may accompany sexual abuse in order to frighten the victim into maintaining silence.

Possible signs of sexual abuse include bruising around the perineal area, complaints of abdominal pain, or reoccurring yeast or urinary tract infections. The patient may also exhibit depression or increased anxiety or anger.

Procedures if a nursing aide suspects that a member of the patient's family is abusing the patient.

It is the obligation of the health care facility to report any incidences of abuse to the state in order to protect the victim and remove him from the situation.

The nursing aide should be vigilant for any signs of abuse and should report any signs of abuse to the charge nurse. This includes any physical signs of abuse, any statements made by the patient regarding abuse, or any signs of neglect. Once the findings have been reported to the charge nurse, the health care team will determine if any abuse has taken place and notify the proper authorities. The nursing aide should not try to discuss the subject with the victim by herself, and she should not attempt to confront or accuse the abuser.

*Nursing aide procedures if she becomes frustrated:* In many cases of abuse, the caregiver is responsible for inflicting the abuse on the patient. The abusive behavior may stem from feelings of exhaustion or frustration related to caring for another person. Nursing aides can also feel this type of frustration. Whenever a nursing aide finds herself becoming frustrated with a person or situation, she should remove herself from the situation as quickly as possible. She should take a moment to try and recognize the source of her frustration. She might find it helpful to talk to the charge nurse about her feelings or try to work with a different team of patients on her next shift. If these measures do not work, it would be beneficial for the nursing aide to seek counseling through her job, to protect herself and her patients.

*What a nursing aide should do if a patient offers her a tip for her services:* In some cases, the patient may attempt to give the nursing aide a tip for her services by offering money or small gifts. The nursing aide should politely and firmly refuse these offers. She should explain to the patient that he is being charged by the health care facility for all services that are provided, and the nursing aide's pay is included in that fee. Usually, one refusal is enough to satisfy the patient. If the patient persists, the nursing aide should remain firm and continue to politely refuse any offers of gifts.

## Certified Nursing Aide Role

A nursing aide is a valuable member of the health care team. Her primary role is to assist the nurse in providing care for the patient. The nursing aide's primary responsibility is to see to the patient's basic needs.

The requirements to become certified as a nursing aide vary depending upon the state. However, most states require a minimum of 75 hours of training, including classroom instruction and review of basic skills. After the training has been completed, a nursing aide must undergo the state certification exam in order to be qualified to provide care to patients. The test is typically divided into two parts, a written exam and a demonstration of skills.

## Continuing Education Importance

Unless a nursing aide continues to study and learn, her skills will become outdated.

The health care facility is required to provide at least 12 hours of continuing education every year in order for the nursing aide to keep her skills up to date.

Continuing education includes teaching regarding new skills and a review of skills that are already known. It is the responsibility of the nursing aide to provide proof of continuing education in order to maintain certification. If the facility does not offer it, the nursing aide should speak to her supervisor about what she can do to acquire her continuing education hours.

## Health Care Team

The health care team is a group of people who provide care for a patient. It includes the patient, the physician, the nurse and other members of the nursing team, and any specialists who may be brought in to aid in caring for the patient.

The patient is the most important member of the health care team; he consents to any treatments that might be performed and must actively participate in order for treatment to be successful. The physician diagnoses any diseases or conditions the patient may have and prescribes medications and treatments to treat the patient. The nurse is responsible for assessing the patient and administering medications. The nursing aide aids the nurse in providing care to the patient. Specialists may be consulted to aid in the patient's treatment, such as a physical therapist or a speech therapist.

## Patient Room Set-Up

It is important for a patient's room to be properly set up prior to his arrival. This ensures the admission process goes as smoothly as possible. When the nursing aide receives word of an admission, she should make sure the room is set up as soon as possible.

The bed linens should be turned down. There should be a clean hospital gown in the room in case the patient arrives wearing street clothes or a soiled gown. The room supplies should be stocked. Telemetry equipment and other necessary equipment should be at bedside; this can include a thermometer, sphygmomanometer, or pulse oximetry probe. Miscellaneous equipment, such as oxygen tubing, Foley catheter equipment, a graduated cylinder, and suction equipment should be provided if it is ordered. The nursing aide should also have the packet of admission paperwork at the bedside.

## Job Interview

A job interview is the first opportunity for a prospective employer to meet an interviewee. It is important to create a good first impression. The interviewee's clothes should be neat and pressed. Female interviewees should wear a skirt or slacks and a blouse. Any makeup should be carefully done so that it is not too heavy. Female applicants should also avoid wearing too much jewelry.

Male applicants should wear a dress shirt and slacks. Shoes should be polished and not scuffed. Nails should be neatly trimmed, and hair should be well groomed.

Topics to Discuss During a Job Interview

A job interview is a time for an interviewer to meet an applicant, but it is also a good time for an applicant to get to know the interviewer and the place in which she will be working.

Before the interview, the nursing aide should think of questions regarding the job description and the facility and write them down. This might include questions about the nurse/patient ratio and the most common types of patients that receive care at the facility. It might also include the number of nursing aides the facility employs and what the turnover rate is. She should avoid asking questions about pay and benefits until after the job offer has been made.

*Forms to Bring to a Job Interview*

When going to an interview, a prospective nursing aide should be prepared. She should have a copy of the questions that she plans to ask during the interview. She should bring a copy of her resume, preferably printed on fine-quality paper stock. She should have a copy of her references, in case the prospective employer wants to check them. She should also have any forms that the employer may have requested. All of these things should be kept together using a paperclip and stored in a folder to keep them neat.

## Work Ethic

Work ethic describes how a person works. If a person has a strong work ethic, it means she works hard at her assigned duties. A nursing aide with a strong work ethic endeavors to complete her assigned tasks in a timely manner, to the best of her ability. She works well in a team situation. She behaves in a manner that is courteous and accommodating. She is punctual, both arriving at work on time and performing tasks at the appointed time. A person with a strong work ethic is also reliable, meaning she can be counted on to perform her assigned tasks well without requiring supervision from her charge nurse.

## Nursing Aide Dress While on Duty

Part of behaving in a professional manner is dressing appropriately. Most facilities have a dress code that all employees should follow. The nursing aide should wear scrubs that follow the dress code. The scrubs should be clean and well mended. Though the scrubs need not be pressed, they should be free of wrinkles. Her shoes should be clean and comfortable. The nursing aide should avoid shoes with high heels or open toes. The nursing aide should also wear minimal jewelry and avoid long necklaces, dangling earrings, and rings. She should avoid fragrances and perfumes. The nursing aide should keep her nails trimmed and should avoid wearing nail polish or acrylic nails to work.

## Nursing Aide Responsibilities

The nursing aide's primary responsibility is to care for the patient's basic needs.

- She should see to the patient's nutritional needs by distributing the meal trays and feeding the patient if necessary.
- She should also aid the patient in exercising.
- Whenever necessary, the nursing aide will aid the patient with elimination and hygiene needs.

- 80 -

- The nursing aide may be responsible for checking vital signs, answering call lights, and reporting any changes to the charge nurse.
- There may also be other tasks that will be the nursing aide's responsibility, and these tasks will be detailed by the health care facility.

## Interpersonal Relationships

Good interpersonal relationships are the key to a group of people working as a team. This is necessary in order to provide adequate patient care. A nursing aide can maintain good interpersonal relationships in a number of ways. She can behave with a positive attitude. She should try to avoid gossiping about coworkers and should avoid openly criticizing them. She should perform any tasks assigned to her promptly and should notify the charge nurse if there are any tasks that she is unable to perform during her shift. She should also utilize teamwork by regularly offering to provide assistance to others and thanking them for any assistance provided to her.

## Responsibilities in a Code Situation

In a code situation, it is vital for the health care team to work together in order to provide a positive outcome for the patient. Prior to a code, the nursing aide should be aware of her responsibilities.

She should know the location of the crash cart in case she is asked to retrieve it and how to activate the code system if she discovers a patient who is unresponsive. In a code situation, the nursing aide's primary role will be to obtain any necessary equipment. If she has her CPR certification, the nursing aide may also provide relief CPR. It is important that the nursing aide listen to any instructions provided to her. If the room is crowded, the nursing aide should leave to make sure it does not remain too crowded but should remain near the door so that she can hear any instructions.

## Becoming Ill Prior to Scheduled Shift

A nursing aide should take every precaution to prevent herself from becoming ill. If she becomes ill, she should avoid reporting to work, where she could possibly spread her illness to the patient population. Most health care facilities have policies regarding sudden illness, and the nursing aide should make herself aware of these policies. Most facilities require the nursing aide to provide notification of absence at least two hours prior to the start of her shift. It also may be necessary to provide a doctor's excuse if her illness required her to miss multiple days of work.

## Scheduling Conflict

A nursing aide should endeavor to make her supervisor aware of any important events so that the facility might work around those events. However, scheduling conflicts do occasionally occur. Most health care facilities do have policies regarding scheduling conflicts, and the nursing aide should familiarize herself with these policies. If a conflict arises, the nursing aide should talk to her colleagues and try to make arrangements to switch workdays in order to accommodate her schedule. If the nursing aide is unable to find someone to switch with her, she should talk to her supervisor and attempt to make arrangements that can accommodate her schedule. Under no circumstances should the nursing aide not show up for work.

## Refusing an Assignment

A nursing aide must have a valid reason to refuse an assignment. There are a number of reasons why she might do so. A particular assignment might not be part of a nursing aide's scope of practice.

The nursing aide might feel uncomfortable with the assignment as a result of not knowing how to perform a task or may feel it is unethical or illegal. The nursing aide may refuse an assignment if she feels performing the task will cause harm to the patient or may place herself in danger if she were to perform that task.

<u>Refusing an Assignment</u>

A nursing aide should only refuse an assignment if she has a good reason to do so. After the assignments have been made, the nursing aide should talk to the charge nurse privately about her discomfort regarding the assignment. She should do so in a calm manner. She should explain her concerns and the reason why she is declining the assignment. The nursing aide and the charge nurse should come to an accord regarding the assignment. If the nursing aide and the charge nurse are unable to come to an agreement, the nursing aide should clearly state that she is declining the assignment.

## Patient's Family Participation

In some cases, a member of the patient's family may express a desire to participate in the patient's care. If a family member makes this request, the nursing aide should notify the charge nurse. Ultimately, the decision about allowing the family member to assist with care depends upon the patient as a result of his right to privacy. It may be appropriate in some cases, such as if the patient were going home soon and would require assistance at home.

The nurse should provide instructions to the family member, but the nursing aide should be vigilant while the family member is providing care to ensure that it is being properly done.

## Delegation

Delegation refers to assigning a task to another person. It is within the nurse's scope of practice to assign tasks to the nursing aide; however, it is not within the nursing aide's scope of practice to assign tasks to others. Though the nursing aide is responsible for performing the task, it is the responsibility of the nurse to make sure that it is done properly and in a timely manner. When assigned a task, the nursing aide should make sure she understands how to perform that task. If she does not know how to do it, the nursing aide should either ask for instructions in order to perform the task safely or decline the assignment.

<u>Five Rights of Delegation</u>

It is important for a nursing aide to understand how a task is delegated in order to know if it is being delegated appropriately. The five rights of delegation can be utilized to determine if the assignment is appropriate.

1. The first right refers to the task: whether the task can be delegated to another person or if it is more appropriate for it to be performed by the nurse.
2. The second right refers to the circumstance; the nursing aide should ask herself if the patient is stable enough for the task to be safely performed.
3. The third right refers to the right person. The nursing aide should ask herself if she feels she is able to perform the task appropriately.
4. The fourth right refers to directions. The nursing aide should ask herself if she received adequate instructions regarding the assignment.
5. The final right refers to supervision. The nursing aide should ask herself if she is going to have an appropriate amount of supervision while performing the task.

# Disease Process

## Hospice Care

Hospice care is a series of services that are available to provide end-of-life care for patients with terminal illnesses. Hospice care is typically made available to patients with a life expectancy of six months or less. A patient can receive hospice care at home, in a hospital, or in an extended-care setting. The purpose of hospice care is to help the dying patient to pass with dignity, while controlling pain and other symptoms and making the patient comfortable. The patient is cared for medically, while receiving spiritual and psychological support. Similar emotional support is provided to family members of the patient.

## Stages of Grief

When a patient is informed that he is going to die, he typically undergoes five stages of grief. These stages can occur in any order prior to acceptance, and the amount of time spent in each stage is dependent upon the patient. The first stage is denial. The patient is unable or unwilling to accept that he is going to die and often claims that a mistake has been made. The next step is anger. The patient is unable to deny the illness and reacts with resentment and anger. The following step is bargaining. The patient attempts to make a deal with a higher power in order to prolong life. Depression is the next step as the patient realizes that bargaining will not work to undo the situation. The final stage is acceptance as the patient realizes the situation and begins to make end-of-life preparations.

> **Review Video: Patient Treatment and Grief**
> Visit mometrix.com/academy and enter code: 648794

## Priorities in Caring for a Dying Patient

If a patient is actively dying, there are a number of priorities that should be kept in mind while caring for the patient. The patient should be kept as free of pain as possible. If the patient complains of pain, notify the nurse immediately so that the patient can be medicated appropriately. The patient should also be kept as comfortable as possible. Allow him to eat and drink what he wishes. Listen to the patient's concerns, and give emotional support to both the patient and the family. Allow the family to remain at bedside. Keep in mind that, even if the patient appears to be comatose, the sense of hearing is the last sense to fade prior to death.

### Patient Care

Patient care should be provided as often as needed for a patient who is dying. The patient should be kept clean; if the patient needs to be bathed while the family is in the room, the family should be asked to step out while patient care is being performed. The only exception is if the patient asks certain members to stay or if his culture requires him to be bathed by family members. Oral care should be provided every two hours and as needed. If excessive oral secretions build up, the patient's nurse should be notified so the mouth can be suctioned gently. The patient should be turned every two hours. Vital signs are typically not ordered on a patient who is dying.

### Signs and Symptoms of Impending Death

When death is imminent, the patient will experience a significant change in vital signs. The heart rate will become slow and irregular and will feel thready when palpated. The patient's respiratory rhythm will become shallower, with the breaths becoming infrequent. The breathing may take on a rattling quality that results from mucous in the respiratory tract; this is referred to as a death rattle. Blood pressure and temperature will decrease. As a result of the diminished vital signs, the patient will become unarousable. Death typically occurs within minutes after the blood pressure is lost.

*Providing support to grieving family members:* If the family is not present when the patient dies, the nurse aide should make an effort to make the body look presentable prior to the arrival of the family.

The body should be placed in a supine position and covered with a blanket up to the chest. If necessary, a clean gown should be placed on the body. The family should be given as much time as they need to view the body. The nurse aide should make an effort to offer comfort to the family, listening to them and providing emotional support where needed. The nurse aide should offer the family anything they might need, such as tissues or water. While viewing the body, the family should be afforded privacy by closing the curtain and shutting the door.

## Postmortem Care

Postmortem care is the process of preparing a body to be taken to the morgue. The nurse aide should make sure to treat the body with the utmost respect.

Ensure privacy by pulling the curtain, wash your hands, and don a pair of gloves. If the patient has dentures, place them in his mouth. Close the patient's eyes. Wash the body as if performing a complete bed bath before dressing the patient in a clean gown. Place a pad over the perineal area. Remove any tubes and lines, and place a dressing over the line insertion sites to prevent oozing. If the facility policy calls for it, shroud the body in a sheet. Place the body in a plastic body bag by tucking it underneath in a manner similar to changing an occupied bed. Close the bag, tie the zippers shut, and slide the body onto a morgue cart using the assistance of one other colleague.

## Rigor Mortis

Rigor mortis is the stiffening of muscles that occurs after death, making the limbs very difficult to move. It typically occurs within a few hours after death and can last up to 72 hours after the time of death. It results from the breaking down of muscle tissue, releasing chemicals within the muscle that cause it to stiffen.

Rigor mortis is significant because the patient's body can get 'stuck' if left in a certain position after death. For this reason, it is important to place the patient in a supine position as soon as possible after death. Certain facility policies call for loosely binding the patient's hands during postmortem care to prevent the limbs from freezing in unusual positions.

> **Review Video: Rigor Mortis**
> Visit mometrix.com/academy and enter code: 220350

## Maslow's Hierarchy of Needs

A need is something that a person requires in order to maintain physical or mental well-being. Abraham Maslow determined the different levels of need that a person requires and organized them on a pyramid diagram.

- The first categories of need are physiological. These are the things a person requires in order to maintain life, such as food, water, and shelter.
- The next level is composed of those needs that pertain to safety and security. These are things a person requires in order to feel safe and comfortable in his environment.
- The next level is composed of love and belonging needs, which meet the person's desire to be loved and accepted as a member of a group.
- Self-esteem needs make up the next level of the hierarchy. These are the things a person needs in order to feel good about himself. The final level of needs includes those required for self-actualization, those things needed for a person to reach his full position.

# Older Adult Growth

## Restorative Care

Restorative care is given to an elderly patient to prepare him for meeting self-care needs after discharge. It is typically provided to patients who have been in the hospital for an extended period of time, such as after breaking a bone or emergent surgery. The type of activities provided during restorative care depends upon individual patient needs.

- Restorative care commonly focuses upon activities of daily living, including physical therapy, nutrition therapy, and occupational therapy.
- Emotional support is also provided to the patient to help treat the anxiety and depression that typically accompanies an extended hospital stay.

## Home Health Care

Home health care is a service provided to patients who are healthy enough to go home but still require the services of a health care provider. The type of home health care provided is dependent upon the patient's needs.

Services that may be provided to a patient by a visiting nurse aide may include assisting with daily hygiene, helping the patient to get dressed, cooking meals, feeding the patient, or range of motion. A nurse aide may provide other assistance, such as changing dressings, shopping for food, or taking vital signs.

## Signs and Symptoms of Dehydration

Dehydration is a life-threatening condition that occurs when the body does not have enough water to perform normal body functions. Patients who are dehydrated may present with sunken eyes and dry mucous membranes. Dehydrated patients will often complain of generalized weakness and constant thirst. Their skin may lose its elasticity as a result of dehydration. They may have a weak, rapid pulse and a low blood pressure. The urine will become darker and more concentrated when patients are dehydrated; a result of the kidneys conserving as much water as possible.

### Encouraging Fluids

If a patient is dehydrated, he must increase the amount of fluids that he consumes in order to restore fluid balance.

Explain to the patient why it is important to consume more fluids, and make sure a water pitcher and glass is within reach. Fluids should be encouraged each time you go into the patient's room. Also, make other fluids available, such as fruit juice or decaffeinated tea or coffee. Try to avoid sugary sodas or caffeinated beverages as these may not quench the patient's thirst. If the patient has family present, ask them to also encourage the patient to drink more.

## Dehydration

Dehydration can be caused by too little intake or too much output.

Limited intake may result if the patient is unable to take in fluid as a result of chronic nausea or difficulty swallowing. The patient may be unable to obtain an adequate amount of fluid if he is confused or kept NPO. Dehydration may also result if the patient is excreting too much fluid.

> **Review Video: Dehydration**
> Visit mometrix.com/academy and enter code: 283651

The most common cause of over-excretion of fluid is frequent diarrhea.

Excessive sweating from fever or exercise may also result in excessive fluid loss. Blood loss after surgery or a hemorrhage or fluid loss after a burn may also cause dehydration.

## Fluid Overload

If a patient is suspected to be in fluid overload, he should be monitored closely. The most significant sign of fluid overload is increased respiratory distress or crackles in the bases of the lungs. The patient may experience edema in the extremities, puffiness around the eyes, or fluid accumulation (ascites) in the abdomen. As the fluid accumulates, the patient may have an unexplained weight gain over a short period of time. A patient in fluid overload may have a bounding pulse, hypertension, or bulging veins. If any of these signs are noticed, the nurse should be notified immediately.

*Causes of fluid overload:* Fluid overload can be caused by excessive fluid intake or by previous medical conditions. Excessive fluid intake can occur if the patient is receiving too much IV fluid or is taking in too much oral intake. The patient's intake and output balance should be closely monitored to ensure the patient does not continue to take in too much fluid. Sodium intake should be monitored as well as too much salt may cause an increased fluid absorption by the kidneys, resulting in fluid overload.

Certain medical conditions, such as heart attack or heart failure, place the patient at an increased risk of fluid overload as the heart may not be able to accommodate an increased amount of fluid. Patients with a history of kidney failure may not be able to effectively compensate for fluid overload and should be closely monitored.

## Constipation

Constipation occurs when the patient's stool is too dry and hard to be able to be passed easily, making him unable to have a bowel movement. The feces become dry and hard as a result of too much water being absorbed from the stool due to poor gastrointestinal motility. If the constipation is not treated, the patient may develop a bowel obstruction.

## Diarrhea

Diarrhea refers to the frequent passage of loose or watery stools. Diarrhea places the patient at risk for developing dehydration because of the amount of fluid lost with the stool. Electrolytes are passed along with the fluid, which can lead to life-threatening electrolyte imbalances if not properly corrected.

- 87 -

<u>Caring for a Patient</u>

Patients who experience multiple bouts of diarrhea are at a significant risk for developing dehydration. They should be closely monitored for any signs or symptoms of dehydration. The number of stools and amount of fluid that are passed should be monitored. A stool specimen should be collected as soon as possible to determine the cause of the diarrhea. If the patient is having frequent diarrhea, it is important to encourage him to drink fluids to prevent him from becoming dehydrated. If his diet allows, the patient should be encouraged to drink two glasses of fluid for every bout of diarrhea. Proper hand hygiene should also be encouraged.

## Constipated Patient Care

During hospitalization, there is a strong risk that the patient will develop constipation. This is often the result of decreased activity and the administration of medications that reduce gastrointestinal motility. The patient's bowel habits should be closely monitored.

If the patient is using a bedpan, the consistency, color, and amount of stool should be noted after every bowel movement. If the patient is able to go to the bathroom without assistance, the nurse aide should inquire about the quality and frequency of the patient's stools. If the patient is constipated, it is important to encourage fluids to prevent drying of the stool. Warm liquids and juices are particularly effective in improving gastrointestinal motility. Caffeinated beverages should be avoided. Foods that are high in fiber should also be encouraged.

## Urinary Tract Infection

The primary symptom of a urinary tract infection is painful or difficult urination.

- The patient may exhibit cloudy urine, which may have a strong or foul smell.
- The patient may experience the need to urinate frequently or may have sudden urgency in the need to urinate.
- The patient may also complain of flank pain or pressure in the pelvis.
- The patient may show signs of a generalized infection, such as an elevated temperature, flushed skin, or malaise.
- An elderly patient may also show signs of confusion as a result of the infection.

<u>Prevention</u>

There are a number of ways that a urinary tract infection can be prevented.

If a patient's diet tolerates it, oral fluids should be encouraged. Cranberry juice is particularly helpful in preventing urinary tract infections because it raises the acidity of the urine.

If the patient needs assistance to void, help him to the bathroom as soon as possible as holding in urine can increase the patient's risk for developing an infection. While performing perineal care, the nurse aide should make sure to wash female patients from front to back. If the patient is able to ambulate, showers should be encouraged rather than baths.

## Air Mattress and an Egg Crate Mattress

Pressure ulcers typically develop when the patient is unable to move as a result of illness or injury. As the patient lies in bed, his weight causes breakdown over bony prominences, such as over the shoulder blades and coccyx.

- When inflated, an air mattress decreases the amount of pressure placed upon the bony prominences.
- An egg crate mattress is a foam cushion that has alternating raised areas and grooves that decrease the area of pressure on bony prominences.

Though these items do not replace turning the patient, they can aid in preventing pressure sores in high-risk patients.

## Pressure Sores Prevention

There are a number of methods available to prevent the formation of pressure sores. The primary method of prevention is frequent repositioning. The patient should be turned and repositioned at least every two hours to prevent skin breakdown. Pillows may be used to provide additional support. The patient's feet should be elevated to prevent breakdown on the ankles, and the head of the bed should be kept at less than a 30-degree angle to reduce pressure on the buttocks. The patient's skin should be assessed frequently. The patient's nutritional status should be closely monitored as well since patients who have poor nutrition are at an increased risk of developing a pressure sore.

*How pressure sores are treated:* Pressure sores are difficult to heal as a result of the patient's compromised health status. If a patient develops a pressure sore, it is important to ensure it does not get worse by frequently turning and repositioning the patient. The patient should be placed on a support surface, such as an air mattress. This helps to decrease the amount of pressure on bony prominences. The skin over the affected area should be kept clean and dry. Dressings can be applied to the pressure sore, though the type of dressing depends on the severity of the pressure ulcer. It is also important to ensure the patient maintains good nutrition to ensure healing.

## Patient with Contractures

There are a number of treatment options for a patient with contractures. When a patient first develops a contracture, the nurse and the physical therapist should be notified. Attempts should be made to mobilize the joint using range-of-motion techniques. Heat therapy may be used prior to initiating activity to ease pain and increase flexibility. In some cases, the affected joint may be placed in a splint, which will continuously stretch the joint. Care of the splint should be performed as ordered by the doctor. If the contracture does not respond to other treatments, the patient may be taken to surgery to manipulate the tendon.

## Edema

Edema can develop in the patient's extremities as a result of fluid overload or inactivity. The nurse aide can prevent swelling by encouraging the patient to move. If the patient is unable to walk, range-of-motion exercises should be frequently performed. While in bed or in the chair, the patient's legs should be elevated on pillows to prevent swelling in the lower extremities. Massaging the patient's extremities using lotion can also prevent edema. If the patient has a history of heart or kidney failure, his fluid and sodium intake should be closely monitored as too much can result in increased edema.

## DVT and Causes

A DVT, or deep vein thrombosis, is a blood clot that develops in the larger veins in an extremity. DVTs most commonly form in the legs, though the risk of developing a DVT in the arms does increase if the patient has an intravenous line.

DVTs are most commonly caused by immobilization, though other factors such as obesity, infection, tobacco use, and advanced age can increase the patient's risk for developing a clot. The most common signs of a DVT include swelling and redness of the affected extremity. The patient may also complain of pain in the affected extremity.

## Anti-Embolism Stockings

Anti-embolism stockings or T.E.D. hose are tight elastic stockings that are applied to the patient's legs. They are typically prescribed for patients who have undergone surgery or have decreased activity. When a patient is unable to move; blood pools in the legs which increases the risk of developing blood clots and edema.

Anti-embolism stockings work by placing pressure on the legs, which encourages blood flow. With improved circulation in the lower extremities, the patient's risk for developing a blood clot or edema is decreased. Care should be taken to frequently monitor circulation in the patient's legs while the anti-embolism stockings are in place.

## SCD

A sequential compression device (SCD) is a pair of cuffs that are placed on the patient's legs to prevent the formation of blood clots. While the SCDs are on, the device applies pressure to different parts of the legs over time.

The increased pressure encourages blood flow within the legs, preventing blood clots. Care should be taken while the SCDs are in place to ensure the tubing does not become kinked as this prevents the SCDs from working. The circulation in the patient's feet should also be monitored. Frequent skin care should be performed as the skin underneath the cuffs can become damp and hot.

## Self-Care Program

The purpose of a self-care program is to teach the patient how to provide self care after a long hospitalization or a debilitating illness.

The focus of a self-care program may vary depending on the patient's areas of weakness. For example, a patient who has had a stroke and has weakness on one side of the body must be taught how to perform self-care activities safely and effectively. Self-care programs may include physical therapy, occupational therapy, and nutritional therapy. The patient may also receive assistance with medication management, food preparation, and other activities necessary to live within the community.

## Clock Method of Feeding a Patient

The clock method is a way of describing the placement of food on a plate to a visually impaired patient who is able to feed himself. The patient should be instructed to picture the plate as a clock face, with positions of food located at corresponding numbers. For example, the meat can be at the 12 o'clock position, the vegetables at the 3 o'clock position, bread at the 6 o'clock position, and the fruit at the 9 o'clock position. The nurse aide should try to repeat this pattern at every meal so that the patient is familiar with the locations of each type of food.

## Bowel and Bladder Program

A bowel and bladder program focuses on giving the patient as much control over his bladder and bowels as possible. The purpose is to prevent incontinence by educating the patient on his bowel and bladder habits.

Initially, the nurse aide should note the patient's voiding pattern in order to plan the patient's routine properly. The nurse aide should assist the patient in making note of the amount of food and fluid he takes in and help the patient to the bathroom at regular intervals. By establishing and reinforcing a pattern, the patient is less likely to be incontinent.

## Aspiration Precautions

Aspiration precautions are steps that are taken when a patient has difficulty swallowing to prevent food and drink from going into the lungs. Prior to being fed, the patient should be positioned with the head of the bed at a 90-degree angle. The nursing aide should check to make sure the patient's food and drink is thickened to the prescribed consistency. The patient should be fed slowly, with the nursing aide offering small amounts of food on a spoon. The patient should be allowed an adequate amount of time to chew and swallow. After the meal has been completed, the patient should remain upright for at least a half-hour to prevent reflux. After a half-hour has passed, the patient can be repositioned for comfort.

## Vomiting in Bed

If the patient begins to vomit while lying in bed the nursing aide should act quickly to make sure the patient does not aspirate on the emesis. The patient should immediately be turned on his side. A basin should be provided to catch any emesis. If there is a suction catheter, use it to clean any vomit from the patient's mouth. After the patient is done vomiting, allow the patient to stay on his side until he has recovered. Rinse the patient's mouth and face with cool water, and change the linens if necessary.

# STNA Practice Test

1. When performing a bed bath, what temperature should the water be?

    a. 70-80 degrees Fahrenheit
    b. 105-115 degrees Fahrenheit
    c. 130-140 degrees Fahrenheit
    d. 155-165 degrees Fahrenheit

2. Which of the following tasks is NOT completed during a routine bed bath for a diabetic?

    a. Changing the linens
    b. Inspection and cleansing of skin
    c. Perineal care
    d. Nail care

3. How would you classify a pressure sore that has a pink wound bed, but does not extend through the full thickness of the skin?

    a. Stage I
    b. Stage II
    c. Stage III
    d. Stage IV

4. A patient is scheduled for surgery later in the day. What type of food would you expect on his breakfast tray?

    a. No tray – the patient is NPO
    b. Jell-O and chicken broth
    c. Scrambled eggs
    d. French toast and fruit

5. How can a STNA help prevent the development of pressure sores?

    a. Turning the patient every four hours
    b. Providing a full bed bath three times a day
    c. Doing partial baths every time a patient soils herself
    d. Reducing the amount of fluids the patient drinks to minimize incontinence

6. When is it acceptable for a STNA to wash her hands using an alcohol-based hand sanitizer instead of soap and water?

    a. Before eating
    b. After performing peri care on a patient
    c. After using the bathroom
    d. Between checking on patients

7. A STNA is providing care for a patient on contact precautions. What type of personal protective equipment should she be using?

    a. Respirator
    b. Mask
    c. Gown
    d. All of the above

8. Before entering a patient's room, personal protective equipment (PPE) should be put on in which order?

    a. Gown, mask, gloves
    b. Gown, gloves, mask
    c. Mask, gown, gloves
    d. Mask, gloves, gown

9. When changing linens in an isolation room, which of the following is an appropriate measure to prevent contamination of clean materials?

    a. Placing dirty linens in a plastic bag inside of the patient's room, and then putting the plastic bag into a bag outside of the room that is held open by a second STNA
    b. Shaking out soiled linens to remove solid material before washing
    c. Piling soiled linens outside of the dirty utility room to avoid mixing them with non-contaminated linens
    d. Moving the soiled linens to the dirty utility room before hand washing

10. Which of the following items requires cleaning with a disinfectant prior to use?

    a. Stethoscope
    b. Scalpel
    c. Thermometer
    d. Blood pressure cuff

11. What is the proper term for an infection that is transmitted during a medical procedure?

    a. Droplet
    b. Iatrogenic
    c. Direct oral contact
    d. Fecal-oral transmission

12. For a patient on fall precautions, what is the minimum number of side rails that should be raised while the patient is in bed?

    a. 1
    b. 2
    c. 3
    d. 4

13. Before transferring a patient from the bed to a wheelchair, what is the very first thing the STNA should do?

    a. Place her arms under the patient's axilla and assist her to a standing position
    b. Assist the patient to a sitting position
    c. Allow the patient to dangle her legs for a few minutes before standing
    d. Ensure the wheels on both the wheelchair and the bed are locked

14. What type of assistance would be required for an elderly woman who fell recently, but is still able to ambulate?

    a. Stand by assistance
    b. Minimum assistance
    c. Contact guard assistance
    d. Maximum assistance

15. Which technique is MOST appropriate for a patient with both poor upper body and lower body strength?

    a. Four-point technique
    b. Three-point technique
    c. Swing-to method
    d. Swing-through method

16. A STNA encounters a small fire in a patient's room. The room is empty. What is her first priority?

    a. Rescue patients in the neighboring rooms.
    b. Activate the fire alarm.
    c. Close all fire doors.
    d. Grab a fire extinguisher and attempt to extinguish the fire.

17. Which of the following procedures is NOT appropriate for a patient who has been ordered to be placed in restraints?

    a. Offer toileting and water every one to two hours
    b. Check the patient at least every 30 minutes to ensure there is proper circulation where the restraints are applied
    c. Tie the restraints directly to the bed frame
    d. Tie the restraints directly to the side rails

18. How should a STNA clean an indwelling catheter?

    a. By using a gentle back and forth motion
    b. By using a circular motion towards the body
    c. By using a circular motion away from the body
    d. By using an up and down motion

19. Before taking a meal tray into a patient's room, what should a STNA do?

    a. Record the amount of food/liquids on the intake/output form
    b. Assess a patient's ability to swallow properly
    c. Put on gloves
    d. Ensure that the correct food is on the tray

20. If a STNA notices that a patient appears to be having difficulty swallowing, what should she do?

    a. Notify the nurse immediately
    b. Mash up the food and continue feeding the patient
    c. Give the patient smaller amounts of food with each bite
    d. Nothing; the doctor checked the patient's swallowing already

21. How often should anti-embolism stockings be removed?

    a. Every 4 hours
    b. Every 8 hours
    c. Every 12 hours
    d. Every 24 hours

22. There is a note on a patient's chart that she should be placed in the Sim's position. How should the patient be positioned?

    a. Lying on the stomach with the head turned to the side
    b. On her back with the head of the bed raised to a 90 degree angle
    c. On her back with the head of the bed raised to a 45 degree angle
    d. On her left side with the top leg flexed and supported by a pillow

23. What is the first step for a STNA who is about to put on sterile gloves?

    a. Use the dominant hand to grasp the glove at the cuff and slide it on to the non-dominant hand
    b. Use the non-dominant hand to grasp the glove under the cuff and slide it on to the dominant hand
    c. Wash and dry hands thoroughly
    d. Put on gloves to open the packaging

24. Which of the following is a measurement of the pressure in a patient's heart during contraction?

    a. Systolic blood pressure
    b. Diastolic blood pressure
    c. Apical pulse
    d. Pulse oximetry

25. Which of the following abnormal vital signs should be immediately reported to the nurse?

    a. Oral temperature of 99.2 degrees
    b. Respiratory rate of 5
    c. Blood pressure of 126/72
    d. Pulse rate of 59

26. Which fluids should be included in the measurement of a patient's intake?

    a. 8 oz. of milk
    b. 250 mL of intravenous fluid
    c. 6 oz. of Jell-O
    d. All of the above

27. What is the first thing a STNA should do when measuring a patient's height and weight?

    a. Wash her hands
    b. Verify the patient's identity by inspecting her armband
    c. Allow the patient's legs to dangle for a few moments before allowing her to stand up
    d. Assist the patient with ambulation to the scale

28. Which of the following is an example of subjective data?

    a. The patient has a pulse rate of 88 bpm
    b. The patient states that she has a pain level of 8
    c. The STNA notes that the patient has flushed cheeks
    d. The STNA notes that the patient has cloudy urine

29. While completing her documentation, a STNA notices that she made a mistake while writing in a patient's blood pressure. How should she correct the notation?

    a. Use correction fluid to cover the mistake

    b. Scribble out the incorrect number and write the correct number next to it

    c. Draw a single line through the incorrect notation, and write "error," along with her initials. The correct number should be written next to it

    d. Erase the incorrect notation; documentation is always completed using a pencil

30. A patient with which of the following conditions is MOST at risk for dehydration?

    a. Diarrhea

    b. Liver disease

    c. Heart disease

    d. Pneumonia

31. When caring for a patient with diarrhea, which of the following should be recorded in the patient's chart?

    a. Odor of the stool

    b. Types and amounts of fluids the patient is drinking

    c. Number of stools

    d. All of the above

32. How often should a patient who is lying on an egg crate or an inflatable mattress be turned?

    a. Never – patients shouldn't be turned when they are lying on inflatable mattresses

    b. Every 12 hours

    c. Every 6 hours

    d. Every 2 hours

33. Which of the following is NOT an intervention a STNA can use to manage edema?

    a. Elevate the affected extremity.

    b. Use ice or a cold pack to reduce swelling.

    c. Massage the affected extremity using lotion.

    d. Encourage activity or use range of motion exercises.

34. A patient with a shuffling gait, difficulty swallowing and speaking, and short-term memory loss MOST likely has:

    a. Alzheimer's disease

    b. Dementia

    c. Parkinson's disease

    d. Sundowner's syndrome

35. A STNA is caring for a patient with Sundowner's syndrome. Which of the following symptoms should he be especially aware of?

    a. Worsening confusion at night

    b. Risk for falls

    c. Aggression

    d. Difficulty swallowing

36. What is one technique a STNA can use to help a patient with aphasia?

    a. Providing a time limit for the patient to respond

    b. Speaking for the patient

    c. Using a picture or letter board

    d. Giving the patient a pen

37. A STNA is caring for a patient who is becoming agitated. How should she speak to the patient?

    a. In an assertive and confident manner

    b. Not at all; the patient's family members or other staff should interact with the patient

    c. She should not acknowledge the inappropriate behavior and carry on as normal

    d. Calmly and clearly, while attempting to determine why the patient is agitated

38. Hospice care is appropriate for patients who:

    a. are expected to live less than three months

    b. are expected to live less than six months

    c. are actively dying

    d. have been diagnosed with a terminal disease, regardless of their clinical condition

39. Which of the following answer choices correctly lists the five stages of grief in order of their expected occurrence?

    a. Denial, anger, bargaining, depression, acceptance

    b. Anger, denial, depression, bargaining, acceptance

    c. Depression, denial, anger, bargaining, acceptance

    d. Bargaining, denial, anger, depression, acceptance

40. Unless otherwise ordered, how often should a STNA record the vital signs of a patient who is actively dying? The patient has a signed DNR order in place.

    a. Every 5 minutes

    b. Every 15 minutes

    c. Every hour

    d. Never

41. While you are caring for a Buddhist patient, he mentions an upcoming fast day when he can only eat at predetermined times during the day. What is an appropriate response?

    a. Acknowledge his beliefs but explain that you can't make any changes to the facility's dining times

    b. Suggest that his family bring some food from home

    c. Speak with him to determine what his needs will be that day and coordinate with the dining and food team

    d. Apologize for not being able to help him that day

42. When caring for a Jewish patient who observes the Kosher laws, the STNA notices his dinner plate has a dish with pork in it. What should the STNA do?

    a. Bring him the food tray and see if he requests a change

    b. Call the dining/food department to order a new tray, and explain the delay to the patient

    c. Remove the pork from his plate and serve him the tray

    d. Switch trays with another patient

43. What needs are found on the bottom level (most basic) of Maslow's pyramid?

 a. Physiological
 b. Safety/security
 c. Love and belonging
 d. Self-esteem

44. A STNA needs to speak with a patient about the quality and amount of stool he passed that day. How can the STNA help the patient feel more comfortable about disclosing the needed information?

 a. Ask the patient in his room when visitors are present
 b. Ask the patient in the privacy of his room in a quiet tone
 c. Ask the patient in an indirect way and hope the patient understands what the STNA is trying to ask
 d. Ask the patient closed-ended questions

45. A patient states that she is depressed. Which of the following responses by the STNA involves the use of reflection?

 a. I'm sorry that you're feeling depressed
 b. Why are you feeling depressed? Your recovery is moving along well
 c. Do you want to speak with someone about this?
 d. You feel depressed?

46. A STNA is stocking shelves outside a patient's room when the call bell rings. The STNA is not responsible for the patient's care that day. How should the STNA respond?

 a. Ignoring the call bell until the patient's assigned STNA responds
 b. Getting the assigned STNA to check on the patient
 c. Checking on the patient right away to see what she needs
 d. Checking on the patient after stocking the shelves

47. A patient has rung the call bell for the sixth time during the first two hours of a STNA's shift. How should she respond?

 a. Ignore the bell
 b. Call the nurse manager
 c. Remove the bell from the patient's reach
 d. Reassure the patient she will be checked on frequently

48. A STNA has been assigned to care for a ventilated patient, which she has never done before. How should she handle the situation?

 a. Notify the nurse manager that she is not sure how to care for the patient, and request additional instructions or training materials.
 b. Do the best she can while caring for the patient
 c. Speak with the other STNAs to find out what additional care is needed for the patient
 d. Request to switch patients with another STNA

49. A STNA has to ask a sensitive question to a patient who doesn't speak English. How should she ask the question?

 a. Using the patient's family to translate
 b. Calling the hospital's official translation service
 c. Gesturing to the patient in the hope she will understand
 d. Looking up relevant words on the Internet before speaking with the patient

50. A patient's family asks how he is doing after his scheduled MRI. How should the STNA respond?

    a. He had an MRI today?

    b. His MRI results are back. Everything is normal

    c. He seems to be in good spirits. Let me see if he's ready to visit with you and I'll find his nurse to talk to you about the results

    d. Good. He should be ready to go home soon

51. HIPAA guarantees a patient's right to:

    a. confidentiality

    b. informed consent

    c. see their chart

    d. continuity of care

52. A patient has a few questions about the consent forms she signed for a scheduled invasive procedure. How should the STNA respond?

    a. Answer the questions to the best of her ability

    b. Tell the patient that she will ask the nurse to contact the doctor

    c. Tell the patient that she will have plenty of time to ask the doctor before the procedure

    d. Remind the patient that she signed the consent and that the procedure has already been scheduled

53. A family member gives a copy of a patient's advanced directives to a STNA. The patient is scheduled for a minor procedure the next day. Which of the following is an appropriate response?

    a. Tell them to hold onto the copies until and unless they are needed

    b. Tell the family that they are not necessary because the patient is having a minor surgical procedure

    c. Put the copy in the chart

    d. Immediately notify the nurse that the family has advanced directives for the patient

54. A patient is refusing to be turned and it has been several hours since he was last turned. The patient is alert and oriented. How should the STNA respond?

    a. Turn him anyway; he needs it to prevent skin breakdown

    b. Inform him that she will tell the doctor he is refusing care so he can go home

    c. Inform him of the associated risks, and then respect his decision if he still does not want to be turned

    d. Tell him whatever is necessary to obtain his consent to be turned

55. Which of the following would NOT be included in a list of patient responsibilities?

    a. Honesty

    b. Polite and respectful behavior

    c. Maintain all personal property

    d. Compliance with treatment plan

56. A nurse asks a STNA to give Tylenol to a patient who has a headache. The nurse is very busy with another critical patient. What should the STNA do?

   a. Administer the Tylenol; the nurse did the assessment and delegated this task to her
   b. Refuse to give the patient any medication – it is not within her scope of practice
   c. Find the Tylenol and repeat the order – including the patient's name, room number, and instructions – back to the nurse to confirm her directions
   d. Ask another nurse to give the medication

57. While in an elevator, another STNA asks you about the MRI results for the patient in room 307. The STNA cared for the patient while on another unit. What is an appropriate response?

   a. Refuse to answer the question; the STNA is no longer an active member of the patient's health care team
   b. Answer the question fully and honestly
   c. Answer the question without using any identifying information so the others in the elevator won't know who you are talking about
   d. Wait until the other people exit the elevator to answer the question

58. A patient who was injured while committing a criminal act has a right to treatment under which of the following patient rights?

   a. Right to freedom of choice
   b. Right to respectful care
   c. Right to continuity of care
   d. Right of refusal

59. A patient demands to see his medical chart. The STNA should:

   a. give the patient his chart and leave the room to give him privacy
   b. give the patient the chart and stay in the room to ensure he doesn't make any changes
   c. make photocopies of the chart and give them to the patient
   d. inform him that he will need to notify the medical records department to make arrangements

60. A doctor writes a DNR order to:

   a. prevent any care from being provided to a patient
   b. explain the care the doctor feels would most benefit a patient
   c. explain what type of emergency care a patient wishes to have
   d. discharge a patient into hospice care

61. If a patient refuses a treatment and the STNA attempts to perform it anyway, what could the STNA be charged with?

   a. Assault
   b. Battery
   c. Either A or B
   d. Neither A nor B

62. A STNA who forgets to lock the wheels on a wheelchair (which results in a subsequent fall) could be charged with:

   a. assault
   b. battery
   c. malpractice
   d. negligence

63. If a STNA observes the nursing supervisor acting in a negligent way, what should she do?

    a. Speak with the doctor in charge of the patient
    b. Follow the institution's chain of command to determine who to report the behavior to
    c. Go to the institution's president of nursing to report the behavior
    d. Confront the nursing supervisor directly

64. If a STNA begins to suspect that a patient is being abused by a family member, what should she do?

    a. Report it to the charge nurse
    b. Report it to the police
    c. Ignore it because the nurse and doctor probably suspect it too
    d. Confront the suspected abuser

65. Who is the most important member of the health care team?

    a. The nurse
    b. The patient
    c. The physician
    d. The STNA

66. What is the minimum number of hours of continuing education that a STNA should complete each year?

    a. 6
    b. 12
    c. 20
    d. 50

67. What is the BEST way for a STNA to assist during a code?

    a. Administer emergency medications according to the physician's instructions
    b. Document the events
    c. Speak with the family and answer their questions about what is happening
    d. Retrieve emergency equipment, including the code cart or intubation box, and carry out other assigned tasks that fall within a STNA's scope of practice

68. A patient's daughter is requesting to perform morning care for her mother. The patient is okay with the request, and it has been cleared with the charge nurse. What should the STNA do?

    a. Refuse to let the daughter assist
    b. Allow her to perform the morning care and leave the room to provide privacy
    c. Allow her to assist with morning care, but stay in the room to ensure it is being done correctly
    d. Request that the nurse supervise the patient's daughter

69. When the STNA is informed of an admission, what is her responsibility?

    a. Prepare the room, including the linens, gowns, and other necessary equipment
    b. Complete the admissions interview
    c. Make sure the patient's medications have been received from the pharmacy and are correct.
    d. Coordinate the patient's care with the rest of the treatment team

70. Which of the following is NOT a reason for a STNA to refuse an assignment?

a. The STNA feels the task is unethical
b. Performing the task would cause harm to the STNA
c. The STNA had a serious disagreement with the patient's family the day before
d. The assignment is outside the STNA's scope of practice

# Answer Key and Explanations

1. B: Water for a bed bath should be heated up to approximately 105 to 115 degrees Fahrenheit. Any cooler and the water will cool off too much before the end of the bath, chilling the patient. Any warmer and the water will be too hot, and could potentially burn the patient. Filling the basin should be the last thing you do; gather all other supplies first to minimize the cooling of the water. If you don't have a thermometer to measure the water temperature, make sure it is comfortably warm against your elbow or inner arm.

2. D: You should check with your institution's policies on nail care, but generally speaking, a STNA should not provide nail care to a diabetic patient. Diabetics have impaired circulation to their extremities, which can delay healing and even cause severe damage if the skin is injured. For that reason, only a physician, podiatrist, or other specially trained clinician should perform nail care on a diabetic. Performing perineal care, changing the linens, and inspecting the skin should be done during every full bed bath, usually as part of morning care.

3. B: A stage I pressure sore would appear as a reddened area that does not blanch (turn white) when pressed. A stage II pressure sore involves a partial breakdown of the upper layer of skin, but does not extend all the way through the skin. A stage II pressure ulcer may look like a blister. Stage III and stage IV ulcers extend all the way through the skin. You may see the underlying subcutaneous fat in a stage III ulcer, whereas a stage IV may proceed all the way down to the muscles, tendons, or bones. Make sure to report any skin redness to the nurse so that the skin can be thoroughly assessed.

4. A: A patient who is about to undergo surgery or another procedure requiring an anesthetic should be NPO for a minimum of eight hours before the procedure. If the patient receives a tray, you should double check with the nurse before serving the patient his breakfast. If a procedure is scheduled for later in the day, the anesthesiologist may be okay with the patient eating breakfast.

5. C: A patient who is bedbound or spends a majority of the day lying or sitting down is at risk for developing pressure sores. Preventing pressure sores requires multiple interventions, including: turning the patient every two hours, doing a full bed bath once a day and partial bed baths throughout the day as necessary if the patient is incontinent (partial baths should be done whenever a patient soils himself), increasing the protein content of food, and making sure the patient is hydrated. It is not appropriate to do a full bed bath twice a day. Withholding fluids to prevent incontinence is also inappropriate.

6. D: Alcohol-based sanitizers are a great tool to avoid the comparatively time-consuming process of hand washing, and are appropriate in certain situations. The STNA should wash her hands with soap and water before eating, after using the bathroom, after performing a procedure that involves contact with bodily fluids (such as peri care), and when her hands are visibly soiled. She should also wash her hands periodically throughout the day to remove the buildup of alcohol on the hands. It is perfectly acceptable to use an alcohol-based sanitizer between checking on patients, especially if the STNA is not performing care.

7. C: If a patient is on contact precautions the caretaker must wear a gown and gloves. Using a mask or respirator is not necessary unless the patient is on droplet or airborne precautions.

8. A: When entering the room of a patient on isolation precautions, the STNA should put on the gown first, with the opening in the back. After tying the gown closed at the neck and around the

waist, the mask should be put on next. Lastly, the STNA should put on her gloves, ensuring that the cuff of the gloves is covering the cuff of the gown. When leaving the room, the PPE should be removed in the reverse order: gloves, mask, and gown.

9. A: Anything in the patient's room is considered "contaminated," so when you place the soiled linens into the plastic linen bag, that bag is considered contaminated. The STNA should ask a colleague to hold a second bag open at the doorway and place the contaminated linen bag in it. The second STNA can then put the bag on the floor outside of the room until the first STNA is ready to wash her hands and bring it to the dirty utility room. The soiled linens should never be shaken out because of the risk of contaminating other nearby items.

10. C: Items that require cleaning with a disinfectant are ones that come into contact with a patient's mucus membranes but don't puncture the skin. Thermometers and respiratory equipment are good examples of items that should be disinfected but don't require sterilization. Items such as scalpels that penetrate the skin should be sterilized between patients because of the high risk of contamination. Items such as stethoscopes and blood pressure cuffs that just touch the skin can be cleaned with a mild detergent between uses.

11. B: An infection that is transmitted during a medical procedure is called iatrogenic. Droplet transmission is when bacteria or viruses are released in droplets when a person sneezes or coughs. Direct oral contact is transmission between people when there is direct oral contact, such as kissing or sharing a drinking cup. Fecal-oral contamination is exactly what it sounds like: fecal material contaminates food, usually through poor hand washing or poor food preparation techniques.

12. B: A minimum of two bed rails should be raised when the patient is in bed. Raising four side rails is considered a restraint, and should not be done unless directly ordered by the physician. One raised bed rail leaves an entire side of the bed without any boundaries.

13. D: The very first thing that should be done before transferring a patient is to make sure that the wheels on both the wheelchair and the bed are locked. This prevents falls by preventing movement of the bed or wheelchair as the patient is being transferred. Once the STNA has verified that the wheels are locked, she can help the patient to sit up and allow her to dangle her legs for a few moments. Then, she can help the patient stand up and slide into the wheelchair.

14. C: An elderly woman who has fallen previously is at risk for falling again. However, she is still ambulatory, so the STNA should be within an arm's reach in case the patient becomes unsteady or falls again. This is known as contact guard assistance. Stand by assistance and maximum assistance are inappropriate because they provide too little and too much support, respectively.

15. A: Four-point technique is a great method of crutch walking for patients who have poor upper and lower body strength because it balances out the patient's weight on both arms and the alternating legs. Three-point, swing-to, and swing-through methods are all great for a patient who has good upper body strength because these gaits depend primarily on the arms to keep the patient upright.

16. B: This question can be answered using the acronym R.A.C.E. (rescue, activate alarm, confine the fire, evacuate/extinguish). The STNA should first rescue patients in imminent danger. Because the room is empty, her first priority should be to pull the fire alarm. If the fire is small and contained, she could try to extinguish the fire herself with a fire extinguisher using the P.A.S.S. method (pull the pin, aim at the base of the fire, and sweep side to side). If not, she should start closing fire doors and rescuing patients in neighboring rooms if necessary.

17. D: Whenever a patient is placed in restraints, the STNA should make sure there is an up-to-date order from the physician (within the last 24 hours). The patient should be offered the opportunity to use the bathroom or have a glass of water or food at least every one to two hours. The restraints should be checked at least every thirty minutes to make sure they are not too tight or cutting off circulation to the patient's limbs. The ties should be quick-release knots and the restraints should be tied directly to the bed frame. Restraints should never be tied to the side rails in case they inadvertently fall, which could cause injury to the patient.

18. C: A patient with an indwelling catheter has a higher risk of contracting a urinary tract infection, and so catheter and perineal care is very important. The catheter should be assessed and cleaned frequently. After putting on gloves and explaining what you are going to do, you should use warm water to gently clean the urethra and, using a circular motion away from the body, the catheter. The STNA should never clean upwards or use a back and forth motion because of the potential to introduce bacteria into the urethra. Make sure to dry the catheter and patient, check to make sure there are no kinks in the tubing, and then hang the bag from the bed frame.

19. D: Before taking a meal tray into a patient's room, the STNA should ensure that the tray is labeled with the correct name, room number, and diet. Once she has delivered all of the trays, the STNA can go back and assist patients who need help eating. Ability to swallow should be assessed each time a patient is eating. The STNA should always be alert for signs that the patient isn't swallowing properly. As she is collecting the used food trays, the STNA should document the intake for each patient. This is the best time to see what each patient actually ate.

20. A: Because of the serious risk of aspiration and its complications, the STNA should never continue feeding food to a patient with a suspected swallowing issue. She should immediately stop feeding the patient and notify the nurse. The nurse can inform the doctor and arrange for a swallowing study if necessary, or even change the patient's diet to include soft foods or purées only.

21. B: Anti-embolism stockings should be removed once every eight hours to ensure proper circulation and let the skin breathe. When removing the stockings, the STNA should assess the skin to make sure there are no rashes, skin breakdown, or other concerns. She should also check on the patient's toes to assess blood flow while the stockings are on. If the patient complains of numbness, tingling, or discomfort when wearing the stockings, it should be brought to the nurse's attention immediately.

22. D: Sim's position is when a patient is lying on her side with the top leg flexed towards the chest. Choice A, on her stomach, is called the prone position. Choice B, with the head of the bed raised to a 90 degree angle, is called the High Fowler's position. Choice C, on her back with the head of the bed raised to 45 degrees, is called the Semi-Fowler's position.

23. C: When putting on sterile gloves, the STNA should first wash and dry her hands thoroughly. Then, she should open the packaging, taking care not to touch anything inside. Next, she should pick up the glove for the dominant hand at the cuff using her non-dominant hand and slide it onto the dominant hand. Finally, using the gloved hand, she should pick up the second glove beneath the cuff and slide it onto the non-dominant hand. Once both gloves are on, she can then make adjustments to the fit, taking care to avoid touching anything unsterile.

24. A: Systolic blood pressure, or the top number of the patient's blood pressure, looks at the pressure in the patient's heart during contraction. Diastolic blood pressure, or the lower number, looks at the pressure in the heart during rest. The pulse measures the number of cardiac contractions per minute. Pulse oximetry measures the amount of oxygen in the blood.

25. B: Choices A and D are slightly abnormal and should be reported to the nurse, although it is not necessary to do this immediately. A blood pressure of 126/72 is technically considered abnormal, but can probably be largely attributed to the stress of being in the hospital. It is nothing to be overly concerned about. A respiratory rate of five breaths per minute is very slow, and can indicate impending respiratory failure. The STNA should notify the nurse immediately.

26. D: All of the choices are liquids or melt at room temperature (Jell-O), and should be included in the measurement of a patient's intake. The STNA should also measure the amount of tube feeding (including what is used to flush the tube) and other IV medications or fluids. Total intake should be in ccs or mLs (depending on your institution's policies) and recorded every 24 hours.

27. A: Whenever a STNA enters a patient's room to initiate care or perform a task, she should wash her hands, introduce herself to the patient, and explain what she is going to do. Next, she should identify the patient using the patient's armband and two identifiers. Finally, she can perform the task she came in to do, which in this case is measuring the patient's height and weight.

28. B: Subjective data is anything the patient notes or feels, such as her pain level. Objective data is information that can be measured (such as vital signs) or observed by another person (such as the patient having cloudy urine or flushed cheeks).

29. C: Making documentation errors is common. However, the STNA must understand how to deal with these errors. She should never use correction fluid or scribble out the error so it is illegible. A pencil should never be used for documentation. When an error is made, simply draw a single line through the mistake and place the correction, the word "error," and your initials next to it.

30. A: A patient with diarrhea is at a high risk for dehydration, so all complaints from the patient and direct observations of diarrhea should be reported to the nurse. Signs of dehydration include dry mucus membranes, weakness, and thirst. The STNA may also observe dark urine or sunken eyes. As long as it's not contraindicated, the STNA should encourage the patient to drink extra water to help replace the lost fluids.

31. D: When caring for a patient with diarrhea, it is important to note all of the information in the answer choices in the patient's chart, as it can be vitally important to the care and treatment plan for the patient. Additionally, the doctor will need the information to gauge the severity of the diarrhea and dehydration. The STNA should also note how much fluid is passed with each stool and how often the patient is having episodes of diarrhea.

32. D: Unless the patient is on a special bed that is designed to be used without turning, the patient should always be turned every two hours. Simply adding an egg crate or inflatable mattress to the existing bed is not enough to eliminate or reduce the need to turn the patient. An egg crate can help reduce the pressure on the patient's skin and bony prominences, but the patient should still be turned every two hours.

33. B: True edema is usually a result of poor circulation, so using an ice or cold pack would be of little use in managing it. Useful interventions help stimulate blood flow and blood return. Elevating the extremity will help promote lymphatic drainage and venous return to minimize edema. Movement through ambulation, massage or range of motion exercises are also great ways to treat and minimize edema.

34. C: All of these symptoms are signs of Parkinson's disease. Alzheimer's disease, dementia, and Sundowner's syndrome all produce similar symptoms, which include confusion, agitation, and wandering. A shuffling gait, though, is the hallmark symptom of Parkinson's disease. A patient with

Parkinson's needs special help with ambulation because their gait is so unsteady, and with eating because they frequently have difficulty swallowing their food.

35. A: Patients with Sundowner's syndrome typically have worsening confusion at night. They may become agitated and wander off the unit. During the day, patients with Sundowner's typically aren't as confused. Possible interventions include checking on and reorienting the patient frequently, and preventing day time sleep so that it is easier for the patient to sleep at night. A patient with Sundowner's may also be at risk for falls or aggression or have difficulty swallowing, but these symptoms are secondary to the confusion they experience at night.

36. C: Aphasia is an acquired inability to understand language and express oneself through speech. Patients with aphasia have different levels of ability, and should be approached with patience. Setting a time limit and speaking for the patient are not productive or helpful in terms of helping the patient relearn these skills. A pen and paper may be helpful in some situations, but many patients aren't able to read or write as a result of their aphasia. A picture or letter board is a universal method of communication, and offers an easy way to communicate because it is so simple to use.

37. D: Patients may become agitated for any number of reasons. They might be in pain or be uncomfortable. They could be hungry, thirsty, have to go to the bathroom, or even be bored or scared. Understanding what is causing someone's agitation is the best way to relieve it. The STNA should continue to interact with the patient in a calm, clear, and professional manner. She may need to set boundaries as necessary, especially if the behavior persists.

38. B: Hospice care is appropriate for patients who are expected to live less than six months. Patients who are transferred into hospice care typically sign a DNR order and are treated using pain relief measures.

39. A: The first stage of grief is denial that the event happened or is going to happen. Following that is anger at the situation or people involved. Next is bargaining, in which the sufferer bargains with God (I'll do…… if you make this go away). Depression follows as the person starts to deal with their grief. Finally, the patient begins to accept what has happened and can start to move forward. It's important to keep in mind that not everyone goes through the same steps in a linear and straightforward manner. It's not uncommon for someone to progress through one stage quickly and then get held up at a subsequent stage or even regress back to a prior stage.

40. D: Generally speaking, the STNA should never record the vital signs of a patient with a DNR order in place who is actively dying. The clinical staff, including the STNA, should do everything in their power to make the patient and their family comfortable. The family may want the extra time with their loved one without being interrupted. Additionally, the act of having their vital signs taken may cause pain or discomfort for the patient, both of which should be avoided if possible. If, however, the physician has ordered otherwise, the STNA should defer to the wishes of the physician and nurse.

41. C: A patient's religion plays a huge role in how well a patient is able to heal and cope with their disease. The STNA should advocate for her patient and arrange for meals to be sent up at the designated times. She could also coordinate with the nurse and other staff members to ensure continuity. Having his family bring food from home may be one possibility, but the STNA should first try to make arrangements with the dining department.

42. B: Kosher dietary laws are strict guidelines that people who belong to the Jewish faith must follow. The STNA should be sensitive to that and arrange for another tray to be sent up from the

- 107 -

dining department. It is not appropriate to simply remove the pork from the patient's tray or wait until the patient requests a change. The STNA should not switch his tray with another patient's. Each tray is specially prepared based on patients' nutritional needs and allergies.

43. A: Physiological needs must be met first, and are therefore at the bottom of the pyramid. These needs include food, water, sex, and oxygen. The next level is the need for safety and security. This isn't restricted to just physical security, but also the safety of one's family, morals, finances, employment, and property. Love and belonging (usually to a group such as a family or friends) is the next level. The final two levels are self-esteem (encompassing self-confidence and achievement) followed by self-actualization, which includes creativity, spontaneity, and morality.

44. B: When speaking with a patient about sensitive topics, it can be helpful to ask the patient when he is alone and use a quiet, sensitive tone. The STNA should be direct, however, and avoid using clichés or euphemisms. It can also be helpful to use open-ended questions, which gives patients the opportunity to answer for themselves.

45. D: Reflection is the process of listening to what patients say and reflecting it back to them, giving them an opportunity to further explain what they meant. This is the technique used in Choice d. Choice A is an example of showing empathy. Choice B is not helpful for the patient; they may be feeling depressed for reasons that are entirely unrelated to their illness. The response is not sensitive to the patient's needs. Choice C may be appropriate, but shuts down the conversation and the relationship between the patient and the STNA.

46. C: Because of the potential for a patient emergency, it is never appropriate for a STNA to ignore a call bell. She should respond to the bell and see if she is able to assist the patient. Stocking the shelves is not a priority, especially when it comes to patient care. It may be necessary for the STNA to get the assigned aid to help with patient care, but she should verify that nothing urgent is needed first.

47. D: The STNA should never ignore a patient's call bell because it could potentially alert the staff to a dangerous situation. That doesn't mean, however, that the patient has a right to abuse the staff and call bell system. The STNA should establish clear boundaries and expectations about when it is okay to use the call bell. She should also understand that it is quite likely that the patient is anxious or lonely, and should agree to check on her at established intervals. This may help alleviate some of the anxiety. The nurse manager may need to get involved if the above interventions aren't successful.

48. A: The STNA should never take on a patient or task that she does not feel sufficiently trained to handle or comfortable with. She should immediately speak privately with the nurse manager to request additional instructions or training. The STNA should never "just do the best she can" because of the potential for serious complications. Colleagues may be an additional source of information, but the nurse manager should be immediately made aware of the situation, and should be the primary point of contact for the STNA.

49. B: When a sensitive topic is involved, the STNA should utilize the hospital's translation system. This can help the patient feel more comfortable and answer the question more appropriately and accurately. Family members are a good source of assistance for routine tasks and matters that don't involve sensitive topics. Gesturing to the patient in the hope she will understand the question is not a great technique because it can easily lead to misunderstanding. Looking up words on the Internet can be helpful, but will not guarantee that either the patient or the STNA will understand what the other is trying to say.

50. C: Unless the family member has a legal document stating that they are the patient's guardian or holds power of attorney, the patient has a right to privacy. Further, the STNA should not give results to any patient or family member. It's fine to say that the patient seems to be feeling well and offer to get the nurse to discuss details about the test.

51. A: HIPAA guarantees a patient's confidentiality and privacy. It also requires healthcare providers to provide patients with a list of policies that have been designed to protect their privacy. Only providers who are directly caring for someone should have access to their medical chart.

52. B: A STNA should not discuss procedures or what was in the consent forms the patient signed. Only a physician can review and inform a patient of the risks and benefits of having a procedure or treatment. A patient can always withdraw their consent, even if they're about to go into the procedure room. The nurse should notify the physician that the patient has questions so he can arrange to see the patient and discuss her concerns.

53. D: Advanced directives should be promptly placed in the patient's chart and the nurse or physician should be notified. They may need to verify the orders or write new orders for the hospital's order system. Everyone involved in the care of the patient needs to be on the same page and aware of the patient's wishes, even if they are only having a minor procedure.

54. C: A patient has the right to refuse a procedure, even if doing so is not in his best interest. The STNA should explain why frequent turning is important and what may happen if he continues to refuse. Asking what the patient is concerned about or why he doesn't want to be turned can be helpful in identifying solvable problems. If the patient still refuses, the STNA should notify the nurse, who can also speak with the patient and document the incident in the chart.

55. C: All of the choices with the exception of maintenance of personal property are patient responsibilities. Valuable items should be returned to the patient's home or stored with hospital security. Patients should be honest with their caregivers and act in a respectful and appropriate manner. While a patient has the right to refuse treatment, it is expected that they will work with the care team to develop and maintain a mutually acceptable treatment plan.

56. B: A STNA should never administer medication; it's not within her scope of practice. The STNA should go back to the patient and explain that the nurse is with a critical patient and will be with her as soon as possible. Asking another nurse to administer the medication is not an appropriate action because the STNA is then accepting responsibility for delegating the task to another staff member.

57. A: You should refuse to answer the question. The patient has a right to privacy and confidentiality. Even though the colleague cared for the patient in the past, she is not a current, active member of the patient's healthcare team. Therefore, the STNA does not have a right to that information.

58. B: The patient in this situation has a right to respectful care. All patients have the right to receive care, even people injured in the course of committing a crime or those already in the criminal justice system. Patients also have the right to receive care without being discriminated against on the basis of age, gender, nationality, or religion. The right to freedom of choice is the patient's right to have a say in their care plan, and to refuse certain treatments or refuse care altogether.

59. D: A patient absolutely has the right to see his medical chart, but he must follow the procedures put in place by the institution in order to do so. In most cases, the patient will need to contact the

medical records department and submit a formal request in writing. The STNA should not provide copies directly to the patient.

60. C: A DNR order is written for a patient so that the health care team involved in his treatment understands what type of emergency care the patient wishes to have should he become incapacitated. It does not release the physician from providing any care, but simply explains the patient's wishes. For example, the patient may not want to be intubated, but may consent to antibiotics or a feeding tube. In most cases, pain management continues to be an important part of a patient's care, even with a DNR order in place. Often, a DNR order is required for patients entering hospice care, but it is not the only reason why a patient would have such an order.

61. C: A STNA could be charged with assault if she threatens or tries to touch a patient (provide care) without the patient's consent. It does not matter if she actually touches the patient or provides the treatment; the patient just needs to be afraid that she will do it. Battery refers to the actual act of touching the patient in a threatening manner or in a way that the patient has not consented to. In the situation outlined in the question, the STNA could be charged with both assault and/or battery, depending on the specific circumstances surrounding the incident.

62. D: The STNA could be charged with negligence because she performed a task in a way that was inconsistent with her training. Only a professional with advanced training or one who needs to maintain a license, such as a doctor or nurse, can be charged with malpractice. A STNA can't because they only need to maintain a certification, not a license. Assault and battery do not apply because the STNA is not behaving in a threatening manner.

63. B: The STNA should follow the chain of command when determining who to report the behavior to. It is inappropriate to contact the physician in charge of the patient's care because he does not have any authority to deal with this type of nursing situation. It is inappropriate to go directly to the nursing supervisor or president of nursing without following the guidelines set in place by the institution.

64. A: The STNA should immediately report the suspected abuse to the charge nurse so she can determine how best to proceed. It is possible that the suspicions have already been addressed, which is why it is not appropriate to directly report the suspected abuse to the police or confront the potential abuser. The behavior should not be ignored, however, because of the potential for the patient being harmed.

65. B: The most important member of the health care team is the patient. His or her needs—medical, spiritual, and emotional—are the most important. The patient must ultimately consent to and be actively involved in their plan of care. What the physician, nurse, and STNA need, recommend, or want takes a back seat to the needs and wishes of the patient.

66. B: The STNA should complete a minimum of 12 hours of continuing education each year to keep her skills up to date. Additional continuing education hours may be necessary, depending on the skill level and needs of the STNA. Her employer should provide some of the continuing education credits, but it is ultimately the responsibility of the STNA to maintain her certification.

67. D: During a code, the STNA should promptly retrieve emergency equipment or other supplies according to the needs of the physicians and nurses. That may include blood from the blood bank, needles, syringes, etc. Documenting the events and administering medications is the responsibility of the nurse, and is outside the scope of practice of the STNA. The STNA should not answer medical questions from the family, but may be able to provide comfort or support if necessary.

68. C: In cases where the patient will be going home to be cared for by the family, it is definitely appropriate for family members to begin to assist in the patient's care. The STNA should allow the daughter to participate in her mother's care, but should be available to supervise and assist as necessary.

69. A: The STNA should prepare the room, ensuring that linens, personal protective equipment, and other medical supplies are present. The STNA should also help orient the patient to the unit and take vital signs. The nurse should complete the admission interview and assessment and coordinate all aspects of care. This includes contacting the pharmacy and ensuring the correct medications are received.

70. C: A serious disagreement with the patient's family is not a reason to refuse an assignment. The STNA must find a way to work professionally with her patient and the family. If the disagreement begins to interfere with the care the patient is receiving, the STNA should speak with her nurse supervisor about the steps that will need to be taken. The other answer choices are all valid reasons for refusing an assignment.

# How to Overcome Test Anxiety

Just the thought of taking a test is enough to make most people a little nervous. A test is an important event that can have a long-term impact on your future, so it's important to take it seriously and it's natural to feel anxious about performing well. But just because anxiety is normal, that doesn't mean that it's helpful in test taking, or that you should simply accept it as part of your life. Anxiety can have a variety of effects. These effects can be mild, like making you feel slightly nervous, or severe, like blocking your ability to focus or remember even a simple detail.

If you experience test anxiety—whether severe or mild—it's important to know how to beat it. To discover this, first you need to understand what causes test anxiety.

## Causes of Test Anxiety

While we often think of anxiety as an uncontrollable emotional state, it can actually be caused by simple, practical things. One of the most common causes of test anxiety is that a person does not feel adequately prepared for their test. This feeling can be the result of many different issues such as poor study habits or lack of organization, but the most common culprit is time management. Starting to study too late, failing to organize your study time to cover all of the material, or being distracted while you study will mean that you're not well prepared for the test. This may lead to cramming the night before, which will cause you to be physically and mentally exhausted for the test. Poor time management also contributes to feelings of stress, fear, and hopelessness as you realize you are not well prepared but don't know what to do about it.

Other times, test anxiety is not related to your preparation for the test but comes from unresolved fear. This may be a past failure on a test, or poor performance on tests in general. It may come from comparing yourself to others who seem to be performing better or from the stress of living up to expectations. Anxiety may be driven by fears of the future—how failure on this test would affect your educational and career goals. These fears are often completely irrational, but they can still negatively impact your test performance.

> **Review Video:** 3 Reasons You Have Test Anxiety
> Visit mometrix.com/academy and enter code: 428468

# Elements of Test Anxiety

As mentioned earlier, test anxiety is considered to be an emotional state, but it has physical and mental components as well. Sometimes you may not even realize that you are suffering from test anxiety until you notice the physical symptoms. These can include trembling hands, rapid heartbeat, sweating, nausea, and tense muscles. Extreme anxiety may lead to fainting or vomiting. Obviously, any of these symptoms can have a negative impact on testing. It is important to recognize them as soon as they begin to occur so that you can address the problem before it damages your performance.

> **Review Video:** 3 Ways to Tell You Have Test Anxiety
> Visit mometrix.com/academy and enter code: 927847

The mental components of test anxiety include trouble focusing and inability to remember learned information. During a test, your mind is on high alert, which can help you recall information and stay focused for an extended period of time. However, anxiety interferes with your mind's natural processes, causing you to blank out, even on the questions you know well. The strain of testing during anxiety makes it difficult to stay focused, especially on a test that may take several hours. Extreme anxiety can take a huge mental toll, making it difficult not only to recall test information but even to understand the test questions or pull your thoughts together.

> **Review Video:** How Test Anxiety Affects Memory
> Visit mometrix.com/academy and enter code: 609003

# Effects of Test Anxiety

Test anxiety is like a disease—if left untreated, it will get progressively worse. Anxiety leads to poor performance, and this reinforces the feelings of fear and failure, which in turn lead to poor performances on subsequent tests. It can grow from a mild nervousness to a crippling condition. If allowed to progress, test anxiety can have a big impact on your schooling, and consequently on your future.

Test anxiety can spread to other parts of your life. Anxiety on tests can become anxiety in any stressful situation, and blanking on a test can turn into panicking in a job situation. But fortunately, you don't have to let anxiety rule your testing and determine your grades. There are a number of relatively simple steps you can take to move past anxiety and function normally on a test and in the rest of life.

> **Review Video:** How Test Anxiety Impacts Your Grades
> Visit mometrix.com/academy and enter code: 939819

# Physical Steps for Beating Test Anxiety

While test anxiety is a serious problem, the good news is that it can be overcome. It doesn't have to control your ability to think and remember information. While it may take time, you can begin taking steps today to beat anxiety.

Just as your first hint that you may be struggling with anxiety comes from the physical symptoms, the first step to treating it is also physical. Rest is crucial for having a clear, strong mind. If you are tired, it is much easier to give in to anxiety. But if you establish good sleep habits, your body and mind will be ready to perform optimally, without the strain of exhaustion. Additionally, sleeping well helps you to retain information better, so you're more likely to recall the answers when you see the test questions.

Getting good sleep means more than going to bed on time. It's important to allow your brain time to relax. Take study breaks from time to time so it doesn't get overworked, and don't study right before bed. Take time to rest your mind before trying to rest your body, or you may find it difficult to fall asleep.

> **Review Video: The Importance of Sleep for Your Brain**
> Visit mometrix.com/academy and enter code: 319338

Along with sleep, other aspects of physical health are important in preparing for a test. Good nutrition is vital for good brain function. Sugary foods and drinks may give a burst of energy but this burst is followed by a crash, both physically and emotionally. Instead, fuel your body with protein and vitamin-rich foods.

Also, drink plenty of water. Dehydration can lead to headaches and exhaustion, especially if your brain is already under stress from the rigors of the test. Particularly if your test is a long one, drink water during the breaks. And if possible, take an energy-boosting snack to eat between sections.

> **Review Video: How Diet Can Affect your Mood**
> Visit mometrix.com/academy and enter code: 624317

Along with sleep and diet, a third important part of physical health is exercise. Maintaining a steady workout schedule is helpful, but even taking 5-minute study breaks to walk can help get your blood pumping faster and clear your head. Exercise also releases endorphins, which contribute to a positive feeling and can help combat test anxiety.

When you nurture your physical health, you are also contributing to your mental health. If your body is healthy, your mind is much more likely to be healthy as well. So take time to rest, nourish your body with healthy food and water, and get moving as much as possible. Taking these physical steps will make you stronger and more able to take the mental steps necessary to overcome test anxiety.

> **Review Video: How to Stay Healthy and Prevent Test Anxiety**
> Visit mometrix.com/academy and enter code: 877894

# Mental Steps for Beating Test Anxiety

Working on the mental side of test anxiety can be more challenging, but as with the physical side, there are clear steps you can take to overcome it. As mentioned earlier, test anxiety often stems from lack of preparation, so the obvious solution is to prepare for the test. Effective studying may be the most important weapon you have for beating test anxiety, but you can and should employ several other mental tools to combat fear.

First, boost your confidence by reminding yourself of past success—tests or projects that you aced. If you're putting as much effort into preparing for this test as you did for those, there's no reason you should expect to fail here. Work hard to prepare; then trust your preparation.

Second, surround yourself with encouraging people. It can be helpful to find a study group, but be sure that the people you're around will encourage a positive attitude. If you spend time with others who are anxious or cynical, this will only contribute to your own anxiety. Look for others who are motivated to study hard from a desire to succeed, not from a fear of failure.

Third, reward yourself. A test is physically and mentally tiring, even without anxiety, and it can be helpful to have something to look forward to. Plan an activity following the test, regardless of the outcome, such as going to a movie or getting ice cream.

When you are taking the test, if you find yourself beginning to feel anxious, remind yourself that you know the material. Visualize successfully completing the test. Then take a few deep, relaxing breaths and return to it. Work through the questions carefully but with confidence, knowing that you are capable of succeeding.

Developing a healthy mental approach to test taking will also aid in other areas of life. Test anxiety affects more than just the actual test—it can be damaging to your mental health and even contribute to depression. It's important to beat test anxiety before it becomes a problem for more than testing.

> **Review Video: Test Anxiety and Depression**
> Visit mometrix.com/academy and enter code: 904704

# Study Strategy

Being prepared for the test is necessary to combat anxiety, but what does being prepared look like? You may study for hours on end and still not feel prepared. What you need is a strategy for test prep. The next few pages outline our recommended steps to help you plan out and conquer the challenge of preparation.

## Step 1: Scope Out the Test

Learn everything you can about the format (multiple choice, essay, etc.) and what will be on the test. Gather any study materials, course outlines, or sample exams that may be available. Not only will this help you to prepare, but knowing what to expect can help to alleviate test anxiety.

## Step 2: Map Out the Material

Look through the textbook or study guide and make note of how many chapters or sections it has. Then divide these over the time you have. For example, if a book has 15 chapters and you have five days to study, you need to cover three chapters each day. Even better, if you have the time, leave an extra day at the end for overall review after you have gone through the material in depth.

If time is limited, you may need to prioritize the material. Look through it and make note of which sections you think you already have a good grasp on, and which need review. While you are studying, skim quickly through the familiar sections and take more time on the challenging parts. Write out your plan so you don't get lost as you go. Having a written plan also helps you feel more in control of the study, so anxiety is less likely to arise from feeling overwhelmed at the amount to cover.

## Step 3: Gather Your Tools

Decide what study method works best for you. Do you prefer to highlight in the book as you study and then go back over the highlighted portions? Or do you type out notes of the important information? Or is it helpful to make flashcards that you can carry with you? Assemble the pens, index cards, highlighters, post-it notes, and any other materials you may need so you won't be distracted by getting up to find things while you study.

If you're having a hard time retaining the information or organizing your notes, experiment with different methods. For example, try color-coding by subject with colored pens, highlighters, or post-it notes. If you learn better by hearing, try recording yourself reading your notes so you can listen while in the car, working out, or simply sitting at your desk. Ask a friend to quiz you from your flashcards, or try teaching someone the material to solidify it in your mind.

## Step 4: Create Your Environment

It's important to avoid distractions while you study. This includes both the obvious distractions like visitors and the subtle distractions like an uncomfortable chair (or a too-comfortable couch that makes you want to fall asleep). Set up the best study environment possible: good lighting and a comfortable work area. If background music helps you focus, you may want to turn it on, but otherwise keep the room quiet. If you are using a computer to take notes, be sure you don't have any other windows open, especially applications like social media, games, or anything else that could distract you. Silence your phone and turn off notifications. Be sure to keep water close by so you stay hydrated while you study (but avoid unhealthy drinks and snacks).

Also, take into account the best time of day to study. Are you freshest first thing in the morning? Try to set aside some time then to work through the material. Is your mind clearer in the afternoon or evening? Schedule your study session then. Another method is to study at the same time of day that you will take the test, so that your brain gets used to working on the material at that time and will be ready to focus at test time.

### Step 5: Study!

Once you have done all the study preparation, it's time to settle into the actual studying. Sit down, take a few moments to settle your mind so you can focus, and begin to follow your study plan. Don't give in to distractions or let yourself procrastinate. This is your time to prepare so you'll be ready to fearlessly approach the test. Make the most of the time and stay focused.

Of course, you don't want to burn out. If you study too long you may find that you're not retaining the information very well. Take regular study breaks. For example, taking five minutes out of every hour to walk briskly, breathing deeply and swinging your arms, can help your mind stay fresh.

As you get to the end of each chapter or section, it's a good idea to do a quick review. Remind yourself of what you learned and work on any difficult parts. When you feel that you've mastered the material, move on to the next part. At the end of your study session, briefly skim through your notes again.

But while review is helpful, cramming last minute is NOT. If at all possible, work ahead so that you won't need to fit all your study into the last day. Cramming overloads your brain with more information than it can process and retain, and your tired mind may struggle to recall even previously learned information when it is overwhelmed with last-minute study. Also, the urgent nature of cramming and the stress placed on your brain contribute to anxiety. You'll be more likely to go to the test feeling unprepared and having trouble thinking clearly.

So don't cram, and don't stay up late before the test, even just to review your notes at a leisurely pace. Your brain needs rest more than it needs to go over the information again. In fact, plan to finish your studies by noon or early afternoon the day before the test. Give your brain the rest of the day to relax or focus on other things, and get a good night's sleep. Then you will be fresh for the test and better able to recall what you've studied.

### Step 6: Take a practice test

Many courses offer sample tests, either online or in the study materials. This is an excellent resource to check whether you have mastered the material, as well as to prepare for the test format and environment.

Check the test format ahead of time: the number of questions, the type (multiple choice, free response, etc.), and the time limit. Then create a plan for working through them. For example, if you have 30 minutes to take a 60-question test, your limit is 30 seconds per question. Spend less time on the questions you know well so that you can take more time on the difficult ones.

If you have time to take several practice tests, take the first one open book, with no time limit. Work through the questions at your own pace and make sure you fully understand them. Gradually work up to taking a test under test conditions: sit at a desk with all study materials put away and set a timer. Pace yourself to make sure you finish the test with time to spare and go back to check your answers if you have time.

After each test, check your answers. On the questions you missed, be sure you understand why you missed them. Did you misread the question (tests can use tricky wording)? Did you forget the information? Or was it something you hadn't learned? Go back and study any shaky areas that the practice tests reveal.

Taking these tests not only helps with your grade, but also aids in combating test anxiety. If you're already used to the test conditions, you're less likely to worry about it, and working through tests until you're scoring well gives you a confidence boost. Go through the practice tests until you feel comfortable, and then you can go into the test knowing that you're ready for it.

## Test Tips

On test day, you should be confident, knowing that you've prepared well and are ready to answer the questions. But aside from preparation, there are several test day strategies you can employ to maximize your performance.

First, as stated before, get a good night's sleep the night before the test (and for several nights before that, if possible). Go into the test with a fresh, alert mind rather than staying up late to study.

Try not to change too much about your normal routine on the day of the test. It's important to eat a nutritious breakfast, but if you normally don't eat breakfast at all, consider eating just a protein bar. If you're a coffee drinker, go ahead and have your normal coffee. Just make sure you time it so that the caffeine doesn't wear off right in the middle of your test. Avoid sugary beverages, and drink enough water to stay hydrated but not so much that you need a restroom break 10 minutes into the test. If your test isn't first thing in the morning, consider going for a walk or doing a light workout before the test to get your blood flowing.

Allow yourself enough time to get ready, and leave for the test with plenty of time to spare so you won't have the anxiety of scrambling to arrive in time. Another reason to be early is to select a good seat. It's helpful to sit away from doors and windows, which can be distracting. Find a good seat, get out your supplies, and settle your mind before the test begins.

When the test begins, start by going over the instructions carefully, even if you already know what to expect. Make sure you avoid any careless mistakes by following the directions.

Then begin working through the questions, pacing yourself as you've practiced. If you're not sure on an answer, don't spend too much time on it, and don't let it shake your confidence. Either skip it and come back later, or eliminate as many wrong answers as possible and guess among the remaining ones. Don't dwell on these questions as you continue—put them out of your mind and focus on what lies ahead.

Be sure to read all of the answer choices, even if you're sure the first one is the right answer. Sometimes you'll find a better one if you keep reading. But don't second-guess yourself if you do immediately know the answer. Your gut instinct is usually right. Don't let test anxiety rob you of the information you know.

If you have time at the end of the test (and if the test format allows), go back and review your answers. Be cautious about changing any, since your first instinct tends to be correct, but make sure you didn't misread any of the questions or accidentally mark the wrong answer choice. Look over any you skipped and make an educated guess.

At the end, leave the test feeling confident. You've done your best, so don't waste time worrying about your performance or wishing you could change anything. Instead, celebrate the successful completion of this test. And finally, use this test to learn how to deal with anxiety even better next time.

> **Review Video:** 5 Tips to Beat Test Anxiety
> Visit mometrix.com/academy and enter code: 570656

## Important Qualification

Not all anxiety is created equal. If your test anxiety is causing major issues in your life beyond the classroom or testing center, or if you are experiencing troubling physical symptoms related to your anxiety, it may be a sign of a serious physiological or psychological condition. If this sounds like your situation, we strongly encourage you to seek professional help.

# Thank You

We at Mometrix would like to extend our heartfelt thanks to you, our friend and patron, for allowing us to play a part in your journey. It is a privilege to serve people from all walks of life who are unified in their commitment to building the best future they can for themselves.

The preparation you devote to these important testing milestones may be the most valuable educational opportunity you have for making a real difference in your life. We encourage you to put your heart into it—that feeling of succeeding, overcoming, and yes, conquering will be well worth the hours you've invested.

We want to hear your story, your struggles and your successes, and if you see any opportunities for us to improve our materials so we can help others even more effectively in the future, please share that with us as well. **The team at Mometrix would be absolutely thrilled to hear from you!** So please, send us an email (support@mometrix.com) and let's stay in touch.

If you'd like some additional help, check out these other resources we offer for your exam:

http://MometrixFlashcards.com/STNA

# Additional Bonus Material

Due to our efforts to try to keep this book to a manageable length, we've created a link that will give you access to all of your additional bonus material.

Please visit https://www.mometrix.com/bonus948/stna to access the information.